Management of Normal and High Risk Labour During Childbirth

Management of Normal and High Risk Labour During Childbirth

Edited by
Gowri Dorairajan
Professor, JIPMER, Puducherry, India

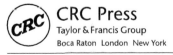

CRC Press
Taylor & Francis Group
Boca Raton London New York

CRC Press is an imprint of the
Taylor & Francis Group, an **informa** business

First edition published 2022
by CRC Press
6000 Broken Sound Parkway NW, Suite 300, Boca Raton, FL 33487-2742

and by CRC Press
4 Park Square, Milton Park, Abingdon, Oxon, OX14 4RN

CRC Press is an imprint of Taylor & Francis Group, LLC

© 2022 Taylor & Francis Group, LLC

Library of Congress Cataloging-in-Publication Data
Names: Dorairajan, Gowri, editor.
Title: Management of normal and high-risk labour during childbirth / edited by Gowri Dorairajan.
Description: First edition | Boca Raton : Taylor & Francis, 2022. | Includes bibliographical references and index.
Identifiers: LCCN 2021062197 (print) | LCCN 2021062198 (ebook) | ISBN 9781032221793 (hardback) |
ISBN 9780367472467 (paperback) | ISBN 9781003034360 (ebook)
Subjects: MESH: Labor, Obstetric | Obstetric Labor Complications | Delivery, Obstetric
Classification: LCC RG525 (print) | LCC RG525 (ebook) | NLM WQ 300 | DDC 618.2—dc23/eng/20220120
LC record available at https://lccn.loc.gov/2021062197
LC ebook record available at https://lccn.loc.gov/2021062198

ISBN: 9781032221793 (hbk)
ISBN: 9780367472467 (pbk)
ISBN: 9781003034360 (ebk)

DOI: 10.1201/9781003034360

Typeset in Times
by codeMantra

Contents

Preface...xi
Acknowledgements xiii
Editor xv
Contributors xvii

Chapter 1   Anatomy of the Pelvis 1

Vandana Mehta

Changes in Pelvis during Evolution 1
Changes in the Pelvis from Infancy to Adulthood 3
True Pelvis: Joints and Ligaments..4
Greater/False Pelvis..5
Lesser Pelvis...5
Pelvic Floor 6
Pelvic Joints and Ligaments 7
Types of Pelvis 10
Sexual Differences in Pelvis...11
Differences in Shape of Female and Male Pelvis...........................12
Pelvic Mechanism 12
References 13

Chapter 2   Understanding the Maternal Passage 15

Gowri Dorairajan

Introduction 15
Clinical Application and Diameter of the Pelvis.............................15
Basic Types of Pelvis..19
Clinical Pelvimetry...22
Suggested Reading 25

Chapter 3   Understanding the Passenger 27

Gowri Dorairajan

Focusing on the Vault 27
Important Landmarks 28
Diameters of the Fetal Skull...29
Summary of the Diameters of Engagement of the Fetus.................29

Chapter 4   Stages of Labour...31

Gowri Dorairajan

First Stage of Labour...31

Chapter 5   Understanding the Power: The Uterine Contractions 37

Gowri Dorairajan

Normal Uterine Contractions 37
Formation of the Uterine Segments..39
References 40

Chapter 6   Understanding the Fetal Journey..41

Gowri Dorairajan

Important Definitions and Terminologies..41
Understanding Fetal Position by Abdominal Examination 44
Mechanism of Labour 46
References 50

Chapter 7   Management of Labour 51

Gowri Dorairajan

Assessment of a Woman in Labour 52
The Management of the First Stage of Labour...................................54
Monitoring of the First Stage of Labour 55
Changing Concepts in the Definition of Active Labour 59
Second Stage of Labour 60
Management of the Third Stage of Labour 63
Episiotomy 64
References 67

Chapter 8   Obstetric Analgesia 69

Chitra Chatterji and Atish Pal

Introduction 69
History..69
Labour Pain and Pain Pathway..70
Techniques of Labour Analgesia 71
Neuraxial Techniques (Epidural and Combined Spinal Epidural) 73
Conclusion..76

Chapter 9   Intrapartum Fetal Surveillance 77

Anish Keepanasseril

Fetal Physiology in Interpretation of the Cardiotocography Findings.....77
Risk Factors of Increased Intrapartum Fetal Compromise.................78
Methods of Intrapartum Surveillance..78
Intrauterine Resuscitation..83
Adjunctive Technologies for Intrapartum Monitoring 83
References 85

Chapter 10 Understanding the Warning Signal of the Uterus and the Fetus.................87

    Gowri Dorairajan

    Predisposing Factors...87
    Clinical Features and Identification of Abnormal Labour.......................89
    Moulding 90
    Caput Succidenum...91
    Synclitism and Asynclitism 91
    References 93

Chapter 11 Abnormal Uterine Contractions 95

    Gowri Dorairajan

    Classification of Abnormal Uterine Contractions 95
    Normal Polarity 97
    Oxytocin 99
    Timeline Definitions for Abnormal Labour...100
    Management Goals of Abnormal Labour... 101
    Complications of Abnormal Labour: Abnormal Labour Can Result in Certain
        Complications Enumerated Below 103
    References 103

Chapter 12 Cephalopelvic Disproportion and Contracted Pelvis 105

    Gowri Dorairajan

    Clinical Identification Tests.. 105
    External Pelvimetry.. 106
    X-ray Pelvimetry 107
    Role of CT Scan and MRI.. 107
    Contracted Pelvis... 107
    Causes for Contracted Pelvis... 108
    Trial of Labour 111
    Management of Trial Labour.. 111
    References 114

Chapter 13 Abnormalities of Second Stage 115

    Gowri Dorairajan

    Arrest in the Second Stage of Labour 115
    Obstructed Labour and Bandl's Ring 121
    Shoulder Dystocia 123
    Delivering Multiple Pregnancies... 126
    Reference.. 128

Chapter 14 Forceps Delivery 129

    Gowri Dorairajan

    Parts of the Forceps 129
    Prerequisites for Forceps Application 131

Types of Application 132
The Procedure.. 132
Forceps Rotation and Extraction 135
References 135

Chapter 15 Ventouse Delivery 137

Gowri Dorairajan

The Apparatus for Ventouse Delivery...................................... 137
Mechanism of Vacuum Assistance 139
Application and Pull... 140
Complications.. 141
Difference in Vacuum and Forceps-Assisted Deliveries 142

Chapter 16 Caesarean Section 143

Gowri Dorairajan

Indications 143
Preoperative Preparations 144
Skin Incision and Steps 145
Difficult Caesarean Section: How to Bail Oneself Out 147
Troubled Situations 152
Elytrotomy.. 153
Postoperative Care... 154
References 155

Chapter 17 Post-Partum Haemorrhage 157

Gowri Dorairajan

Definition.. 157
Clinical Identification 157
Classification 158
Predisposing Factors.. 158
Prevention of PPH 159
References 160

Chapter 18 Clinical Approach to Case of PPH... 161

Gowri Dorairajan

Effective Resuscitation 161
Monitoring after the Initial Management 163
Definitive Management 164
References 167

Chapter 19 Specific Management of PPH... 169

Gowri Dorairajan

Management of Atonic Postpartum Haemorrhage 169
Management of Traumatic PPH 173
Management of Retained Products.. 174
Secondary Postpartum Haemorrhage 175
Massive Blood Transfusion 176
Coagulopathy and Its Management... 177
References 178
Further Reading.. 179

Index.. 181

Preface

Delivering a child is the most humbling experience. The journey of the fetus through the birth canal is the most mysterious. The universal power has filled the unborn fetus and the uterus with innate intelligence. The fetus knows precisely how to steer itself through the birth canal. It is filled with amazing intelligence to adjust and accommodate itself to complete the journey successfully. The uterus is the engine power for this journey and acts as a highly synchronized automated vehicle to complete this journey. Both the fetus and the uterus have a subtle, silent language of expression, more so when the journey appears unfavourable.

Obstetrics has developed as a science to understand this language and the journey. A sound knowledge, a lot of patience, and empathy are necessary to practice obstetrics. In a busy, noisy labour room, it is vital to perceive the silent language of the uterus and the signals communicated by the fetus. A good understanding of the science will give immense confidence and intuitive thinking to the obstetrician who carries a lot of responsibility amongst the uncertainties of the science.

Whereas obstetric practice comprises about three-fourths of all practitioners, only a short duration is spent during the postgraduation period in learning labour management. Slowly, vaginal delivery is becoming a dying art, and caesarean section rates are skyrocketing.

As a hard-core obstetrician and teacher, I feel my moral duty is to impart knowledge and required skills for managing labour to every postgraduate trainee. The practise of obstetrics and childbirth is not just a science but an art. I feel every trainee and obstetrician should experience joy and happiness as they safeguard the fetal journey and uphold the trust and security posed by the labouring woman on them. This book is written for understanding normal labour and abnormal labour with vertex presentation alone. The book has not covered malpresentation or other risk situations and complications due to medical disorders or previous caesarean section.

Acknowledgements

I want to thank my seniors from whom I learnt during the training period. I want to thank women for trusting me with the journey of their unborn child.

I would like to thank all my students for making me feel the need to write a book like this and convert my years of experience into a readable form.

I want to thank my family members for adjusting with me and allowing me to spend a good part of the family time writing the book.

I want to thank the publishers for their timely guidance and patience.

I thank JIPMER and the organizers of the workshop on medical drawing that happened at the right time and helped me draw many diagrams with the software.

I thank the divine force that helped me conceive the book and the unseen power that facilitated me in many silent ways to complete the book.

Editor

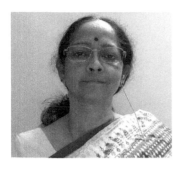

Dr Gowri Dorairajan is a professor and head of a unit at JIPMER, Puducherry, an autonomous National Importance Institution. She is an acclaimed teacher and clinician. She has more than 24 years of teaching experience. In addition, she has vast clinical experience and has worked in many government hospitals with high turnover and deliveries. She did her postgraduation from Lady Hardinge Medical College, New Delhi, from 1992 to 1995 and has vast exposure to various obstetric emergencies and the management of women in labour. She has been working as a professor in JIPMER since June 2013. JIPMER has a high turnover of 18,000 deliveries a year.

She has been a teacher for undergraduates, postgraduates, and DNB trainees and has guided many students with their research work and theses. In addition, she has many ongoing ICMR-funded projects as Principal Investigator. She has more than 70 publications in indexed journals, including international journals. She has presented papers in conferences on more than 45 occasions and regularly visits as faculty to various colleges for postgraduate case discussions.

Labour management is her passion, and she has authored the book *Ruptured Uterus*, published by Springer International, based on her vast experience.

In the era of technology and sub-specialities catching the interest of the trainees and the junior specialists, the author feels that the art of labour management is dying. Therefore, there is a need to impart knowledge about labour management based on understanding the subtle language of the fetus and the uterus. Hence, the author conceived this book.

Contributors

Chitra Chatterji
Transplant and General Anaesthesia
Indraprastha Apollo Hospital
New Delhi, India

Gowri Dorairajan
Department of Obstetrics and Gynaecology
Jawaharlal Institute of Postgraduate Medical
    Education and Research (JIPMER)
Puducherry, India

Anish Keepanasseril
Department of Obstetrics and Gynaecology
Jawaharlal Institute of Postgraduate Medical
    Education and Research (JIPMER)
Pondicherry, India

Vandana Mehta
Department of Anatomy
VMMC & Safdarjung Hospital
New Delhi, India

Atish Pal
Indraprastha Apollo Hospital Sarita Vihar
New Delhi, India

1 Anatomy of the Pelvis

Vandana Mehta
VMMC & Safdarjung Hospital

CHANGES IN PELVIS DURING EVOLUTION

Two unique evolutionary developments in humans are the big size brain and bipedal gait. Due to the advent of hip preservation surgery, morphological changes in hip bone have assumed relevance.

The human hip is an integral part of the anatomic construct with the pelvis and lumbosacral spine. We will compare these evolutionary changes in various species.

Terrestrial vertebrates called tetrapods had four limbs, and in phylogeny, this was considered as a unique change. They are considered descendants of crossopterygians that possessed lobed fins with a narrow attachment. Two adaptations were perceived in response to the terrestrial environment during the evolution of primary amphibians from crossopterygians. The first was the change in position of limb-like paddles for support and locomotion on land. In this regard, forelimbs rotated laterally and hind limbs medially. The second was the articulation of the pelvic girdle with the vertebral column, again a unique feature of tetrapods.

In tetrapods, the pelvic girdle only consisted of endochondral elements, pubis, ilium and ischium, which fused into a single innominate (hip) bone.

Fish

The pelvic fins are attached to the pelvic ring, which lacks attachment to the spine. Hence, it is a "free" element. With the progression of land life, these paired fins develop into limbs to accommodate the weight of the animal against gravity.

It is believed that terrestrial life began with sarcopterygian in the Devonian period some 400 million years ago. Molecular genetic studies have supported the findings that differences between fins and limbs are a result of genetic switches and ensuing minor changes.

In tetrapods as compared to fish, the pelvic ring is not an independent element but attached to the vertebral column by sacral ribs.

Fish developed ventral symphysis, and in tetrapods, distinct ischial and pubic elements were identified.

Reptiles

During evolution, the limbs of the reptiles shifted under the trunk. Although they developed from amphibians, unlike the amphibians, they are not dependent on water to breed. They started to walk in a more upright position. Their front and hind limbs are disposed along the long axis of the trunk and thus are nearer to the body axis. This disposition of the hind limbs modified the hip joint, the proximal end of the femur altered from a cam-like shape in amphibians to a more rotund cam or oval shape. Correspondingly, there were changes in the acetabulum.

Dinosaurs are believed to have developed from reptiles approximately 230 million years ago. The vertical limb position and a rounded hip joint imparted a greater stride length. The acetabular forces were redirected from a medial position in the semi-erect to a dorsal one in the erect posture.

DOI: 10.1201/9781003034360-1

One of the dinosaur hip hallmarks is the "open" acetabulum due to the requirement for a strong bony buttress in the medial acetabular margin.

Bipedal gait became conceivable when the hind limbs were placed under the trunk, relieving the forelimbs for feeding and fighting. Therefore, all carnivorous dinosaurs were bipedal, and a slender and long-tail assisted their balance. In addition, a cylindrical femoral head featured the bipedal dinosaurs, and many species also displayed a femoral neck. Subsequently, the lateral aspect of the neck simulated the greater trochanter.

The hip morphology varies greatly in extent among mammals, and two types of hips are observed. These are the sturdy (coxa recta) and mobile (coxa mobilis or coxa rotunda) hips. The roundness of the femoral head is similar in both these hips, but the junction of the head and neck displays a straight section in coxa recta and a rounded section in coxa rotunda. Hence, there are two positions: "set", which is the position of roundness of the head, and "offset", which is the gap between the head and neck of the femur and the ratio of the thickness of the neck as compared to the head. A low offset characterises the coxa recta while coxa rotunda has a high offset.

The coxa rotunda increases the scope of impingement-free motion within the acetabulum. There is an inversely proportional relationship between the femoral head roundness and offset. Larger mammals have coxa recta, for example, apes that exhibit a rounded femoral head located more symmetrically on the femoral neck along with a higher offset. Earlier, all mammals had a single epiphysis for the greater trochanter and femoral head. This "conjoined" epiphysis resulted in the coxa recta type of hip. However, in other species, including apes, the epiphysis remains separate, one for the greater trochanter and the other for the femoral head [1].

A simple phylogenetic clarification for these hip types is unavailable. Bodyweight plays a role in the extremes of motion. The lightweight mammals like rodents possess coxa rotunda and a distinct ossification pattern. The larger mammals (elephants) have a fused ossification pattern with a rounded femoral head on a thick and vertical neck (neck-shaft angle is 160°). Therefore, when a broad range of hip motion, especially rotation, is required, a "coxa rotunda" and a "separate" ossification pattern is observed, for instance, in apes.

Coxa recta with a low offset is seen where the highest tensile stress is foreseen. On the other hand, coxa rotunda, with a higher offset, raises the range of impingement-free motion within the acetabulum at the cost of tensile strength of the femoral head–neck junction.

Apes

Apes appeared approximately 25 million years ago, characterised by stiff, short backs. Their ilium wings elongated, and the number of lumbar vertebrae reduced to three or four, thereby approximating the rib cage closer to their ilium. Therefore a stiffer "unibody" provided a biomechanical advantage for the larger apes as they were able to climb and swing through trees. Concomitant with a stiff spine, their hips became more mobile, and they were able to climb trees. Moreover, a shallow acetabulum developed with more rounded femoral heads than their quadruped ancestors.

Three exclusive features of man's development from apes are **bipedal gait, encephalisation and elongation of life phases** [2]. Man adopted bipedal gait as the sole mode of transport. Moreover, owing to the increased size of the human head, the birth process had to be contrived, and both these alterations reflected on the pelvis, making it a significant skeletal parameter to study human evolution.

The evolution of bipedal gait led to important modifications in the lumbosacral spine and pelvis. These modifications reflected upon the hip bone and steered significant sex differences in the hips.

Approximately 3 million years ago, the hominid pelvis assumed its shape as is seen in humans today. Functioning abductors and hip kinetics permitted a constant bipedal gait [3]. The human pelvis has a three-dimensional character as compared to the long and flat pelvis of apes.

The ilium curved forwards, thereby relocating gluteus medius and minimus and tensor fascia lata, transforming their role from being extensors in quadrupeds to hip abductors in bipedal walking. The efficiency of these novel abductors is revealed in the bony framework of the femoral neck. Humans have minimal cortical bone on the superior aspect of the femoral neck, whereas apes display a peripheral ring of cortical bone. Since the apes do not possess abductor apparatus, they have a swaying gait. In addition, the compressive forces applied by the anterior gluteal muscles on the superior aspect of the femoral neck negate the tension stresses on this area leading to paucity of cortical bone [4].

The shift to upright posture resulted in a change from a vertical pelvic wall in quadruped mammals to a horizontal pelvic floor in early humans. Likewise, the horizontal abdominal floor of quadrupeds evolved into a vertical abdominal wall in bipeds. Understandably the pelvic floor plays a vital role in the control of continence and reducing the incidence of prolapse in humans [5].

In humans, another important evolutionary development is the attachment of strong sacrospinous ligament and tendinous arch of pelvic fascia to the ischial spines. Childbirth is considered a more unwavering reason for the evolution of the pelvis as compared to bipedal gait.

It is construed that enlargement of the true pelvis led to an increase in brain size in humans. The pelvic diameters of the apes displayed a larger anteroposterior than side to side dimensions. Therefore, the fetus head in apes aligns in the antero-posterior direction.

The ensuing expansion in brain size entailed "intra-pelvic adaptations" at pelvic midplane and outlet levels. The pelvic inlet had already been widened in medial-lateral direction by sacral enlargement.

Biomechanically, the widening of pelvic midplane and outlet mediolaterally spaced out the hip joints, furthermore enhancing the moment arm of body weight, necessitating greater abduction in reparation. Therefore, to maintain an energy-efficient bipedal gait, the femoral neck had to be lengthened.

The enlargement in the pelvic midplane and outlet resulted in forward lengthening of pubic rami and sideway diversion of ischial bones. The latter resulted in an increase in A-P(anteroposterior) direction and the creation of an obtuse subpubic angle.

The ossification in adult humans also deserves special mention as secondary ossification centres do not unite before the end of childbearing age in the third decade.

In humans, this delay in secondary ossification permits continuous lengthening of pubic rami even after growth ceases in the rest of the skeleton [3]. So, the pelvic outlet enlarges in a plane 90° to the largest pelvic inlet diameter.

Consequently, the fetal head rotates 90° through its passage from midplane to outlet. The ischial spines appear as an obstructive feature in the evolution of the pelvis. In quadrupeds, the tail muscles in the ischial spines are of an insubstantial size and are present laterally and dorsally near the sacrum.

In early humans, there was an increase in the size of ischial spines, particularly in the above-mentioned obstructive position of the pelvic midplane. Although they constitute the most menacing bony projections during childbirth, they play a pivotal role in the establishment and resilience of the pelvic diaphragm [6].

In apes, the fetus passes effortlessly through the birth passages, characteristically facing the mother.

In humans, due to rotational birth, the fetus faces away from the mother. This presents difficulty in the airway clearance and removal of the umbilical cord from the neck of the fetus. This disposition of the fetus may result in hyperextension (neck) injuries. Therefore, assisted birth improves the chances of survival in humans [7].

CHANGES IN THE PELVIS FROM INFANCY TO ADULTHOOD

The first year of life experiences a growth spurt in the pelvis. Postnatally, the pelvis increases in length, width and depth as ossification continues. Thereafter from 3 years till puberty, a constant rate of growth is observed. The next stage of growth is at puberty, where an increase in the size of the pelvis contributes to an increase in body size. At birth, the pelvis is ossified partly. The iliac crest, inferior pubic ramus, ischium and acetabulum are unossified at birth.

Two external/bony parameters are used for measuring the growth of the pelvis in children. They are

1. bi-cristal breadth
2. breadth of superior iliac spines.

In the early years of childhood, pelvic height and ilium length may be used as a reference and used as parameters. However, their values alter as the child grows.

Sex differences in the pelvis are determined early in life. External pelvic dimensions are larger in males when compared with females. However, in females, internal dimensions are larger as compared with males.

Ossification

Three primary ossification centres for ilium, pubis and ischium appear around the ninth week, fourth month and fourth to fifth months, respectively. Some parts are still cartilaginous at birth: the iliac crest, the floor of the acetabulum and its inferior margin. The acetabulum is still a cartilaginous cup with a tri-radiate stem extending medially to the pelvic surface as a Y-shaped epiphyseal plate between the three components: ilium, pubis and ischium. The ischium and pubis fuse to form ischio-pubic ramus in seventh or eighth year. Secondary centres of ossification excluding acetabulum develop at puberty and fuse between 15 and 25 years. There are two ossification centres for the iliac crest, one each for ischial tuberosity, anterior inferior iliac spine and the symphyseal surface of the pubic bone. The acetabulum ossifies by three centres between 8 and 9 years of age. The largest centre appears for the anterior acetabular wall fusing later with the pubic bone. The other acetabular centres are for the superior aspect (iliac acetabular cartilage), which fuses with the ilium, and ischial acetabular cartilage, which merges with the ischium. At puberty, these epiphyseal centres enlarge peripherally, thereby accounting for the depth of the acetabulum. Fusion of the acetabular centres occurs between 16 and 18 years.

TRUE PELVIS: JOINTS AND LIGAMENTS

The skeletal pelvis is basically an osseous ring between the two innominate bones and sacrum.

The pelvic girdle is a basin-shaped bony annulus connecting the vertebral column to the two femurs of the lower extremity.

An oblique plane traverses the sacral promontory behind and linea terminalis in front, dividing the pelvis into greater and lesser parts.

The **linea terminalis** comprises the arcuate line of ilium, iliopectineal line and pubic crest.

Clinical anatomy of iliac crest

1. The highest points of the two iliac crests, called the intercristal plane, lie at the fourth lumbar vertebra. Additionally, it marks the preferred site for lumbar puncture (L4-L5).
2. The iliac crest is a common site for bone biopsy using a posterior superior iliac spine landmark.

Pelvic Walls

Anatomically, the pelvis is that part of the body which is enclosed by pelvic girdle.

The word "pelvis" literally means "basin" and resembles a pudding basin with most of the anterior wall being deficient. This is compensated by the lower part of the abdominal wall, where the aponeurotic fibres of the three anterolateral muscles lie in front of the rectus abdominis.

The pelvic brim divides the "false or greater pelvis" above from the "true or lesser pelvis" below.

GREATER/FALSE PELVIS

The greater pelvis is considered a continuation of the abdomen and, therefore, occupied by inferior abdominal viscera (ileum and sigmoid colon). It lies above the linea terminalis and consists of the iliac fossae and sacral base.

LESSER PELVIS

The inferior pelvic girdle provides the skeletal framework for the lesser pelvis and the perineum. Its boundaries are the pelvic surface of hip bones, sacrum and coccyx.

It contains the pelvic organs and is considered a narrow continuation of the greater pelvis. It is of significant obstetric relevance and has a median curved axis. The superior opening of the lesser pelvis is occupied by the viscera in life while the inferior by the pelvic floor and its sphincters.

The lesser or true pelvis has obturator internus, piriformis, levator ani and coccygeus muscles.

The levator ani and coccygeus muscles form the pelvic diaphragm or floor of the pelvis. The superior concave surface of this musculo-fascial pelvic diaphragm forms floor of the true/lesser pelvis, and the inferior concave surface forms the roof of the perineum. The lateral pelvic wall is constituted by the hip bone and the obturator internus with its fascia. The posterior pelvic wall is constituted by the sacrum and piriformis, which passes laterally into the greater sciatic foramen.

Perineum refers to the area of the trunk between the thighs and buttocks containing the anus and external genitalia: penis and scrotum in males and vulva in females.

PELVIC INLET/SUPERIOR PELVIC APERTURE

Pelvic inlet/superior pelvic aperture is referred to as pelvic brim and is impinged by the sacral promontory behind. It is of anthropological and obstetric relevance.

Pelvic Brim

Pelvic brim is the bony rim enclosing the pelvic inlet. It is made of the following structures in continuity:

1. Right and left linea terminalis laterally and in front
2. Sacral ala and promontory behind

Each linea terminalis is comprised of:

1. Pubic crest
2. Pectineal line of the pubis
3. Arcuate line of ilium

Pubic Arch

Pubic arch is the conjoined inferior rami of ischium and pubis of the two sides form the pubic arch. The inferior borders define the subpubic angle. The width of the subpubic angle is ascertained by the distance between right and left ischial tuberosities during a per vaginal examination.

CAVITY OF LESSER PELVIS

The ends of the alimentary canal and urogenital ducts traverse this cavity. It consists of rectum behind and urinary bladder in front in both sexes, and in females, the uterus interposes between the rectum and urinary bladder.

PELVIC OUTLET/INFERIOR PELVIC APERTURE

Pelvic outlet/inferior pelvic aperture is indented behind by sacrum and coccyx and on the sides by ischial tuberosities. There are three main arcs: anteriorly pubic arch, which is formed by the ischio-pubic rami, greater and lesser sciatic notches between ischial tuberosities laterally and sacrum coccyx posteriorly. These notches are converted into foramina by the vertebropelvic ligaments. With these ligaments intact, the shape of the outlet becomes rhomboidal – anterior limbs being the ischio-pubic rami and posterior limbs being the sacrotuberous ligaments and coccyx in the median plane.

PELVIC FLOOR

Pelvic floor is a gutter-shaped muscular sheet; the pelvic diaphragm hangs around the midline viscera – urethra and anal canal in both sexes and in addition the vagina in females (Figure 1.1a).

The pelvic floor muscles are the levator ani and coccygeus. These muscles arise progressively from the body of the pubis, tendinous arch over obturator fascia, ischial spine, inserting into coccyx and the post-anal plate.

The muscles pass downwards and backwards towards the midline from this origin, thereby directing the pelvic floor downwards and forwards.

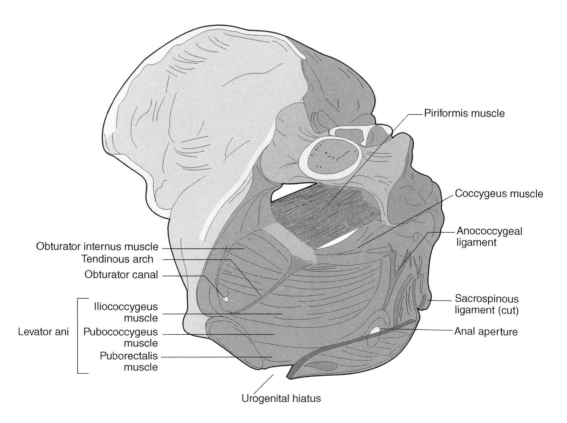

FIGURE 1.1A Lateral view of the pelvis.

ACTIONS OF THE FLOOR MUSCLES

1. Support pelvic viscera retaining them in a normal position.
2. The muscles counteract the raised intra-abdominal pressure as in coughing, sneezing and weight lifting.
3. The pelvic floor relaxes in expulsive efforts. So, in defaecation, the abdominal wall and diaphragm contract while the puborectalis relaxes to straighten the anorectal junction. The floor slopes down to enhance the funnel shape. Similarly, the pubovaginalis fibres of levator ani help the urethral sphincter at the end of micturition in females.
4. The floor plays a vital role in parturition by guiding the fetal head towards the pelvic outlet.

The muscular and fibrous components of the floor are stretched during childbirth rendering it liable to tears.

The diameters of the pelvic inlet, cavity and outlet are discussed in the forthcoming chapter.

PELVIC AXIS AND INCLINATION

In the standing posture, the plane of the brim is oblique, lying at 60° with the horizontal plane, while the plane of the outlet/inferior aperture is about 15°. Since the pelvis tilts forwards, the posterior parts of both planes are above the anterior. In a sitting position, the body weight is borne by the inferiomedial aspect of ischial tuberosities.

ANATOMICAL POSITION OF PELVIS

In an erect person, the anterior superior iliac spine and upper border of pubic symphysis lie in the same vertical plane. The upper border of the pubic symphysis, ischial spine, the tip of coccyx, femoral head and apex of the greater trochanter lie in the same horizontal plane.

This plane traverses the pelvic cavity and coincides with the tip of the clinician's finger during per rectal or per vaginal examination.

The inferior pole of ovaries in females and seminal vesicles in males lie in this plane.

PELVIC JOINTS AND LIGAMENTS

The joints of the pelvis are the sacroiliac, sacrococcygeal and pubic symphysis.

The chief ligaments are the vertebro-pelvic and iliolumbar ligaments (Figure 1.1b and c).

SACROILIAC JOINT

This strong joint has two components: an anterior plane type of synovial articulation connecting the auricular surface of the ilium and sacrum and a posterior syndesmosis between tuberosities of these bones. There is minimal movement at this joint. The sturdiness of the joint contributes to the weight transmission from the vertebral column to the lower extremity. As age advances, this joint becomes partly fibrous, and the articular surfaces fuse.

Ligaments
The sacroiliac ligaments are anterior, interosseous and posterior.

1. Capsular – attached to the articular margins.
2. Anterior sacroiliac ligament – flat band connecting the bones above and below the pelvic brim. It is well developed close to the arcuate line and posterior inferior iliac spine. This ligament is stronger in females producing a characteristic pre-auricular groove in the female ilium.

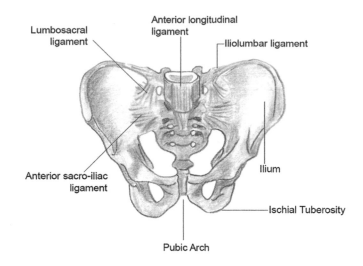

FIGURE 1.1B front view of the pelvis.

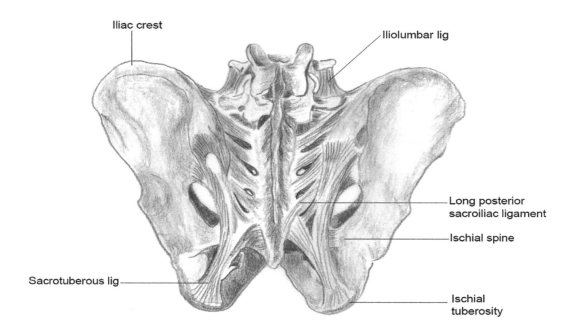

FIGURE 1.1C Posterior view of the pelvis.

3. Interosseous sacroiliac ligament – it is considered the largest typical syndesmosis. It is a very strong extracapsular ligament attaching the sacrum to the ilium behind the joint. It attaches to deep pits on the posterior surface of the lateral sacral mass. The most superficial fibres constitute the posterior sacroiliac ligament. The posterior rami of spinal nerves and vessels pass between interosseous and posterior sacroiliac ligaments.

Sacrotuberous Ligament

Sacrotuberous ligament is a flat band of immense strength; it blends with the posterior sacroiliac ligament and attaches to the posterior border of the ilium, posterior superior and inferior spines and to the transverse tubercles of the sacrum below the auricular surface and upper part of the coccyx. From this extensive attachment, the ligament extends to the medial surface of the ischial tuberosity. A forward prolongation from the ischial attachment of this ligament attaches to a curved bony ridge termed as "falciform process". This ligament is considered to be a remnant or degenerated tendon of the long head of the biceps femoris. It provides attachment to the gluteus maximus on the posterior surface. It is pierced by perforating cutaneous nerves and branches of inferior gluteal vessels and coccygeal nerves.

Sacrospinous Ligament

This ligament is present on the pelvis aspect of the sacrotuberous ligament. Presented with a broad base by which it attaches to the side of the lower part of the sacrum and upper part of the coccyx, it narrows at its apex to attach to the ischial spine. It represents the degenerated part of the coccygeus muscle.

Iliolumbar Ligament

Iliolumbar ligament is a V-shaped ligament, the apex of which attaches to the transverse process of a fifth lumbar vertebra from which two bands diverge – upper band attaching to the iliac crest and a lower band blending with the anterior sacroiliac ligament. The upper band provides attachment to the quadratus lumborum, continuing with the anterior layer of the lumbar fascia.

Functions

The vertebropelvic ligaments resist upward tilting of the lower part of the sacrum under the downward thrust at its upper end. They also convert greater sciatic notches into foramina.

Movements

The minimal anteroposterior rotation occurs around a transverse axis around 5 cm vertically below the sacral promontory. This accompanies flexion and extension of the trunk – this range increases in pregnancy.

Clinical Anatomy

1. Functional aspects

    Most of the movements of the joint are restricted by the irregular articular surfaces to slight gliding and rotation.

    Therefore, ligaments provide the sole stabilising mechanism for the sacroiliac articulation. The transfer of weight from axial skeleton to ilia occurs primarily through the interosseous sacroiliac ligaments and thence to the femora on standing and ischial tuberosities on sitting. The weight of the body conveyed through the fifth lumbar vertebra has a tendency to thrust the sacrum downwards and forwards towards the symphysis. The interosseous sacroiliac and iliolumbar ligaments oppose these gliding movements of the joint surfaces. Similarly, the function of opposing the forward rotation of sacral promontory is performed by sacro-tuberous and sacrospinous ligaments. The sacrospinous ligaments slacken in later months of gestation, allowing minimal rotation of the sacrum.

2. The anaesthetic solution introduced through sacral hiatus into the sacral canal blocks the sacral nerve roots, thereby anaesthetising the birth canal, pelvis and perineum while sparing the lower extremity. This **pudendal nerve block** is utilised to block the pain of episiotomy during labour.

3. The pelvic joints and ligaments slacken in pregnancy concomitant with an increase in the movements. As a result, there is a reduction in sacroiliac articulation effectiveness, allowing rotation and alteration in pelvic diameters. One positive effect is an increase in the transverse diameter facilitating the fetal passage.

    One disadvantage of this weakened locking mechanism of the sacroiliac joint is that it further strains the ligaments.

    Therefore, this sacroiliac subluxation causes pain due to tension in the ligaments after parturition.

SACROCOCCYGEAL JOINT

Sacrococcygeal joint is the symphyseal/secondary cartilaginous joint between the sacral apex and base of coccyx. The joint cavity has an intervening fibrocartilaginous disc. Five sacrococcygeal ligaments unite the articulating surfaces – one anterior, two posterior and two lateral ligaments. The posterior sacrococcygeal ligament has two laminae: deep and superficial. The latter closes over the sacral hiatus. The two lateral sacrococcygeal ligaments attach to the transverse process of the coccyx and inferior sacral angle, providing a passage for the anterior ramus of the fifth sacral nerve.

Only slight flexion and extension occur at this joint.

Clinical Anatomy

In late pregnancy, the ligaments become lax, and there is an increased range of movements, both of which may result in trauma during delivery.

PUBIC SYMPHYSIS

Pubic symphysis is a secondary cartilaginous type of joint whose articulating surfaces are covered by hyaline cartilage with an intervening fibrocartilaginous disc. The joint is reinforced superiorly by the superior pubic ligament and inferiorly by the arcuate pubic ligament.

Arcuate Pubic Ligament

It connects the lower border of the symphyseal surface of pubic bones, extending laterally to attach to the inferior ramus of the pubic bone. It blends superiorly with inter pubic disc. Its base is separated from the anterior border of the urogenital diaphragm by an opening for the deep dorsal vein of the penis/clitoris.

Interpubic Disc

Interpubic disc connects the medial pubic surfaces, each covered by a layer of hyaline cartilage with intervening fibrocartilage.

Movement

Usually, this joint permits no or very minimal movement, although a slight amount of rotation and displacement is possible along with movements at sacroiliac and hip joints. In addition, some separation may occur during parturition.

Clinical Anatomy

Symphysiotomy, the splitting of the pubic symphysis, may be performed to enlarge the birth canal for delivery.

TYPES OF PELVIS

MORPHOLOGICAL CLASSIFICATION OF PELVIS

Classification of pelvis has immense obstetric and forensic implications. The pelvis exhibits sexual and racial variations, and these have anthropological value.

One of the early attempts to classify types of the pelvis was based on shape and utilised the pelvic brim index.

Pelvic brim index = anteroposterior diameter/transverse diameter × 100.

The following types of the pelvis are identified:

1. Platypellic (transversely flat)
2. Mesatipellic (intermediate form)

3. Dolichopellic (anteroposterior long)
4. Brachypellic (android)

The brachypellic type or android pelvis was classified based on anatomical and radiological data and is responsible for severe obstruction in childbirth.

Another classification based on skeletal measurements divides the pelvis into four types:

1. Gynaecoid (Mesatipellic)
2. Android (Brachypellic)
3. Anthropoid (Dolichopellic)
4. Platypelloid (Platypellic)

SEXUAL DIFFERENCES IN PELVIS

The pelvis is one of the important bones of the human body displaying sexual dimorphism. These sexual differences are related to function. Locomotion is the primary function in both sexes. In the females, it is reformed for childbirth.

A broad overview of the sexual differences to the following facts:

1. The female pelvis is broader for smooth passage of the fetal head.
2. Female bones are slenderer as compared to male bones.

The subpubic angle in males is acutely pointed, like a gothic arch, whereas in females, it is rounded like a Roman arch.

Following are the important differences elucidated in male and female pelvis bones.

I. **Pelvic brim**

In males, the sacral promontory indents the outline, and the brim is widest at the back (heart shaped).

In females, the indent caused by sacral promontory is less prominent, so the brim is widest anteriorly (transversely oval).

II. **Ilium**

The male iliac crest is more rugged with an obvious medial inclination anteriorly. In females, it is less curved with more vertical iliac blades and shallower iliac fossae. These features explain for greater prominence of hips in females.

III. **Sacral base**

The articular facet for the fifth lumbar vertebra is more than a third of the total sacral basal width in males and less than a third in females. In addition, females have a broader sacral ala.

IV. **Pubis**

The subpubic arch in males measures $50°–60°$, whereas in females, it is more rounded, measuring $80°–85°$.

V. **Ischio-pubic rami**

In males, there is a roughened everted area for attachment of crura of the penis, whereas in females, it is not everted as the crura of the clitoris is not well developed.

VI. **Ischium**

Ischial spines are closer and inturned in males. The greater sciatic notch is wider in females due to increased backward tilt of sacrum and greater anteroposterior pelvic diameter at lower levels.

VII. **Sacrum**

Curvature – female sacra are less curved, whereas male sacra are more evenly curved.

Sacral index – the sacral index relates sacral breadth with length, and its value is 105% in males and 115% in females.

Auricular surface – smaller and more oblique in females.

Pre-auricular sulcus – more pronounced in females.

Chilotic line – line extending from iliopectineal eminence to nearest point on anterior auricular margin and then to iliac crest. The auricular point divides the chilotic line into two segments: anterior (pelvic) and posterior(sacral), each expressed as a percentage. The chilotic index has reciprocal values in the male and female pelvis – the pelvic part is prominent in females and the sacral part in males.

DIFFERENCES IN SHAPE OF FEMALE AND MALE PELVIS

Females have "coxa profunda" with a deep acetabulum having fovea at or medial to the illio-ischial line. Further, a rounded femoral head with a high head–neck offset characterises the female pelvis.

The coxa recta has a straight segment on its anterosuperior femoral head with its cartilage extending onto a sturdy femoral neck, thereby reducing the head–neck offset. Both these hip types predispose to degenerative changes through femoral acetabular impingement [8].

Properties that characterise the female pelvis maximise the dimensions of the birth canal. Therefore, broadening of the true pelvis sets the acetabulum further apart, increasing the lever arm of body weight on the hips. To some extent, elongation of the femoral neck can compensate for this, lowering the required abdominal work in gait. This femoral neck length is associated with fracture risk [9]. An alternative mechanism for retaining bipedal gait is to place the acetabulum deeper in the Pelvis- Coxa Profunda. Hence the femoral head is rounded in coxa profunda with a good head–neck offset. The femoral neck affects the acetabular rim and labrum when the hip is extended and laterally rotated or flexed and medially rotated [10]. This acetabular rim and labrum damage may result in osteoarthritis usually seen in females in their late 50s and 60s [8].

In males, coxa recta type is observed with aspherical femoral heads and asymmetrical head–neck offset on a thick and short femoral neck. The clinical trait of coxa recta is reduced internal rotation in flexion, becoming painful with years as degenerative changes develop.

In land animals, there was a requirement of larger muscles for support of body weight and necessary thrust to be transmitted through the hind limbs. Therefore, a larger iliac size ensued in these animals and articulation of the innominate bones with the vertebral column.

In conclusion, as compared to the fish family, tetrapods displayed a fusion of the three elements into a single entity that is the innominate bone.

Thus, the pelvis was established by joining the two innominate bones anteriorly by a symphysis and posteriorly with the sacrum at the sacroiliac articulation.

The pelvis subserves not only locomotor function but also transmits stresses between the axial skeleton and lower limbs. Regarded more as an irregular ring rather than a "basin", as its name suggests, it encloses the urogenital organs and allows passage of their external openings.

PELVIC MECHANISM

1. Although primarily concerned with supporting and protecting the viscera, the pelvis distributes the weight from the head, trunk and upper limbs to the lower extremity.
2. In addition, it offers attachment to trunk and leg muscles concerned with posture and locomotion.
3. It provides attachment to the erectile bodies of external genitalia.
4. A vertical trans-acetabular plane divides it into two arches: an anterior and a posterior arch. The anterior arch formed by pubic bones and their superior rami connect the lateral

pillars like a tie beam to avoid separation. This arch also acts as a compression thrust against the medial femoral thrust.

5. The posterior arch consists of the upper three sacral vertebrae and the bony pillars of sacroiliac articulation to acetabular fossae. It is concerned with weight transmission.

REFERENCES

1. Serrat MA, Reno PL, McCollum MA, Meindl RS, Lovejoy CO. Variation in mammalian proximal femoral development: comparative analysis of two distinct ossification patterns. *J Anat.* 2007; 210(3): 249–258.
2. Gibbons A. Anthropology: The birth of childhood. *Science.* 2008; 322(5904): 1040–1043.
3. Lovejoy CO. The natural history of human gait and posture. Part 1. Spine and pelvis. *Gait Posture.* 2005; 21(1): 95–112.
4. Kalmey JK, Lovejoy CO. Collagen fiber orientation in the femoral necks of apes and humans: do their histological structures reflect differences in locomotor loading? *Bone.* 2002 Aug; 31(2): 327–332.
5. Abitbol MM. Effect of posture and locomotion on energy expenditure. *Am J Phys Anthropol.* 1988; 77(2): 191–199.
6. Abitbol MM. Evolution of the ischial spine and of the pelvic floor in the Hominoidea. *Am J Phys Anthropol.* 1988; 75(1): 53–67.
7. Trevathan WR. The evolution of bipedalism and assisted birth. *Medical Anthropol Quarterly.* 1996; 10(2): 287–290.
8. Ganz R, Leunig M, Leunig-Ganz K, Harris WH. The etiology of osteoarthritis of the hip: an integrated mechanical concept. *Clin Orthop Relat Res.* 2008; (466): 264–272.
9. Faulkner KG, Wacker WK, Barden HS, Simonelli C, Burke PK, Ragi S, et al. Femur strength index predicts hip fracture independent of bone density and hip axis length. *Osteoporos Int.* 2006; 17(4): 593–599.
10. Smith-Petersen MN. The classic: Treatment of malum coxae senilis, old slipped upper femoral epiphysis, intrapelvic protrusion of the acetabulum, and coxa plana by means of acetabuloplasty 1936. *Clin Orthop Relat Res.* 2009; (467): 608–615.
11. Lovejoy CO. Evolution of human walking. *Sci Am.* 1988; 259(5): 118–125.

2 Understanding the Maternal Passage

Gowri Dorairajan
Jawaharlal Institute of Postgraduate Medical
Education and Research (JIPMER)

INTRODUCTION

The female pelvis has changed during evolution from quadrupeds to the present *Homo sapiens*, as detailed in Chapter 1. The obstetric aspect of the pelvis needs to be understood at three planes: the inlet of the pelvis, the plane of least pelvic dimensions, and the outlet of the pelvis.

CLINICAL APPLICATION AND DIAMETER OF THE PELVIS

THE INLET

The inlet has the shape of a rounded wedge in such a way that the widest transverse diameter cuts the anterior-posterior diameter not halfway through but a little posterior.

Boundaries of the inlet: The inlet is bound anteriorly by the upper border of the pubic symphysis. It continues along the pubic tubercle, pubic crest, iliopectineal eminence, and pectineal line. It ends posteriorly by the linea terminalis on the ala of the sacrum to the sacral promontory (upper border of the S1 vertebra). This area bounded by the margins is the *plane* of the inlet.

This plane separates the false pelvis above from the true pelvis below.

Axis: A line drawn perpendicular to the plane in its centre is the axis and it would pass through the umbilicus when extended upwards and through the coccyx when extended downwards. Thus, in a normal standing position, the plane of the inlet is at a 55°–60° angle to the horizontal plane.

Diameters of the inlet: This will be discussed as

- The anteroposterior
- The transverse
- The oblique diameters

Antero-posterior Diameter

Three clinically relevant anterior-posterior diameters extend from the pubic symphysis in front to the sacral promontory behind. Let us learn the details of these diameters. These are called *conjugates*. It is important to understand that the pubic symphysis is a biconvex joint and has upper and lower borders and anterior and posterior surfaces.

The anatomical conjugate: Extends from the upper border of the pubic symphysis to the sacral promontory – the anatomical or *true conjugate* measures around 11 cm.

The convexity of the pubic symphysis restricts the use of this diameter by the descending fetus, and the actual diameter available to the fetus is a little smaller, called the *obstetric conjugate (Vera)*. This extends from the centre of the posterior surface of the pubic symphysis to the sacral promontory. It is about 1.5 cm less than the *diagonal conjugate* and measures about 10 cm.

DOI: 10.1201/9781003034360-2

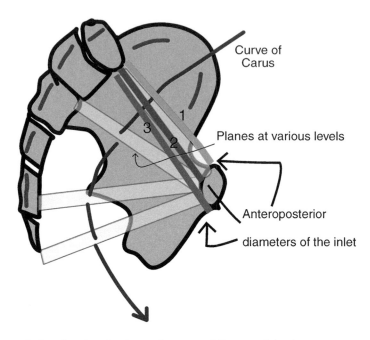

FIGURE 2.1   Lateral view showing the planes, the curve of Carus, and the three anteroposterior diameters of the inlet of the pelvis. 1: Anatomical conjugate; 2: Obstetric conjugate; 3: Diagonal conjugate.

However, when clinical pelvic assessment is done, the fingers are limited by the lower border of the pubic symphysis. Thus, the anterior-posterior diameter that can be measured clinically is from the lower border of the pubic symphysis to the sacral promontory. This is called the *diagonal conjugate* (Figure 2.1). It is, on average, about 12.5 cm.

The width of the pubis symphysis, its inclination to the sacrum, and the inclination of the brim can change the relation of the diagonal and obstetric conjugate.

The anteroposterior anatomical diameter of 11 cm is divided by the transverse diameter at the widest part of the inlet, into 7 cm in front and 4 cm behind, making the inlet a rounded wedge that is wider posteriorly.

Transverse Diameter

It is the dimension across the widest part of the inlet. It measures about 13 cm. It is set a little posterior rather than in the middle of the plane of the inlet. It is exaggerated in the case of platypelloid or flat pelvis.

The oblique diameter of the inlet extends from the same side sacroiliac joint behind to the opposite iliopectineal eminence. Thus, the reference starting point is the sacroiliac joint. Therefore, the right oblique starts from the right sacroiliac joint and extends to the left iliopectineal eminence. This measures around 12 cm.

Sacro-cotyloid Diameter

This is from the midpoint of the sacral promontory to the iliopectineal eminence. The left diameter extends from the sacral promontory to the left eminence. This diameter is used by the fetus in women with a flat pelvis with a reniform brim with an extremely narrow anteroposterior diameter. It is about 9–9.5 cm.

Important points of clinical significance at the inlet of the true pelvis:

- In a gynaecoid pelvis, the inlet is a rounded wedge, and the transverse and the oblique diameter are longer, and the anteroposterior diameter is the shortest.

- The plane of the inlet should form a more than 90° angle with the sacrum. In the android pelvis, this angle is acute.
- The axis of the inlet has a downward and backward direction. During labour, nature ensures that the longitudinal axis of the uterus aligns to the axis of the inlet to push the fetus in the right direction.

Mid Pelvic Cavity

This is the most spacious part and called the plane of greatest pelvic dimensions. This extends from the centre of the posterior surface of the pubic symphysis to the S2-S3 junction posteriorly. It extends on both sides along the obturator foramen anteriorly, the inner surface of the Ilium bone, the sacrosciatic notch, and the soft tissue around them. Therefore, the *transverse diameter* cannot be easily measured or defined as it is restricted by the soft tissue. The line drawn perpendicular to this mid pelvic plane at the level of the anteroposterior diameter is called the axis and is directed downwards. The plane is round and about 12 cm in all three diameters

The conventional mid pelvic contractions are described at the plane of least pelvic dimensions.

The plane of least pelvic dimensions also marks the end of the mid pelvis and upper boundary of the obstetric outlet of the pelvis.

Outlet of the Pelvis

The outlet of the pelvis has two aspects, the obstetric outlet and the anatomical outlet.

The obstetric outlet: It is the segment between the plane of least pelvis dimensions above and the plane of anatomical outlet below.

The plane of least pelvic dimensions: It is bound by the lower border of the symphysis pubis anteriorly, the ischial spines on the side, and extends posteriorly along the sacrospinous ligament to the lower border of the S5 vertebra.

The Diameters

The *anteroposterior diameter* extends from the lower border of the pubic symphysis to the tip of the sacrum (lower border of the S5 vertebra, also called the sacrococcygeal joint).

The imaginary line from the two ischial spines divides the anteroposterior diameter into a posterior segment called the posterior sagittal and anterior segment – the anteroposterior diameter measures around 12 cm and the posterior sagittal diameter is about 5.5 cm.

The transverse diameter extends between the two ischial spines and is the narrowest. It measures about 10.5 cm. The area bound is the plane and the perpendicular line passing through this plane or the axis is directed downwards and forwards.

Anatomical outlet: A lozenge-shaped plane with a triangle in front and back shares a common base. The two triangular areas are set at two different coronal planes. It is bounded by the lower border of the pubic symphysis anteriorly, the inferior ramus of the pubic bones, the ischial tuberosity anterolaterally, and the tip of the coccyx posteriorly.

The common base is at the level of the ischial tuberosities and is also the extent of the *transverse diameter*. It measures about 11 cm (Figure 2.2).

The *anteroposterior diameter* extends from the lower border of the pubic symphysis to the tip of the coccyx. Since the coccyx can move backwards at the sacrococcygeal diameter, this diameter is dynamic and can increase. This is the longest diameter of the outlet, measuring 13 cm. The posterior sagittal diameter of the anatomical outlet extends from the tip of the sacrum to the midpoint of the inter-ischial tuberosity line. It measures about 7–9 cm.

The *oblique diameter* is indistinct and limited by the soft tissues on the sides.

The area bounded by the bony landmarks forms the *plane*, and the perpendicular drawn from its centre or the *axis* has a downward and forward direction.

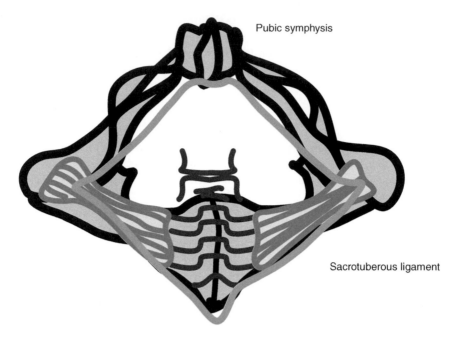

Pubic symphysis

Sacrotuberous ligament

FIGURE 2.2   View showing the anatomical outlet of the pelvis. Blue line represents the border of the outlet, green is the ligament.

The *subpubic angle* is the angle between the two inferior rami of the pubic bone. Normally, this should be obtuse (more than 90°) in a gynaecoid pelvis. The more acute or narrow it is, the more the wasted space of Morris. This makes the fore-space narrow, and the head gets pushed posteriorly to use the space behind. The space between the lower border of the pubic symphysis and the upper edge of the head fitting in the subpubic angle is the space of Morris. The angle can range from 85° to 135°, and on average, it is about 105°.

Curve of Carus

The line joining the axis of the three levels of the pelvis, that is, the inlet, mid pelvic cavity, and the outlet, forms a "J"-shaped curve. The curve initially points backwards and downwards, then downwards, and finally forwards and downwards. The fetal journey follows this direction during labour (Figure 2.1).

The Importance of the Plane of Least Pelvic Dimensions

- It marks the "0" station. The station below this level is taken as plus and above as minus.
- It is the landmark bony point for administering pudendal block.
- It is the plane of least pelvis dimensions and the plane to define mid pelvic contractions.
- Levator ani muscle attaches to the ischial spines.
- Internal rotation of the head during labour occurs at this level.
- It marks the anatomical level of the external os and is used as the reference point for observing the descent of the cervix.
- The curve of Carus changes its direction from backwards to forwards at this level.

The overall depth of the pelvis is an essential aspect during the fetal journey. The typical distance from the sacral promontory to the tip of the sacrum is 9–11 cm and till the tip of the coccyx is 12–14 cm. Therefore, a deeper pelvis can have problems during labour. Similarly, a pubis symphysis longer than 4 cm will increase the pelvis's anterior depth and cause problems.

Having understood the various diameters of significance at the three levels of the pelvis, let us understand the compensatory diameters.

Compensatory Diameters

It is very important to understand the dynamics of the pelvis and the diameters. The reciprocal diameter can compensate for the lack of one diameter.

Brim

At the level of the brim, the anteroposterior diameter, which is the shortest, is compensated by the transverse diameter. The area of the plane of the brim has to be adequate. The anteroposterior × transverse diameter should be more than 120 (the area of the brim more than 95 cm²). The anteroposterior diameter can be measured clinically. The transverse diameter is difficult to measure and requires imaging (Mengert's index and Nicholson's method), but it is indirectly reflected on the intercristal diameter and the distance between the anterior superior iliac spines. If the anteroposterior diameter appears narrow on clinical pelvimetry (described in Chapter 12), then we need to focus on the adequacy of obstetric and anatomical outlet. This will help us to differentiate between a generally small pelvis, android, and flat pelvis. In a flat pelvis, only the anteroposterior diameter of the brim is narrow. Other diameters progressively improve from the inlet to the outlet, and vaginal delivery can be looked forward to without difficulty if the head negotiates the brim.

An oval brim with a long anteroposterior diameter and a deep pelvis are more likely to be associated with posterior positions. In these situations, the adequacy of the pelvis at the plane of least pelvic dimensions becomes important.

Plane of Least Pelvic Dimensions

The transverse diameter at the level of the two ischial spines is the narrowest diameter at this plane. This is also the plane where internal rotation occurs. The posterior sagittal diameter at this plane compensates for the transverse diameter. When the inter-ischial spine diameter is borderline, the focus should be on the sacral curve and the prominence of the sacrococcygeal joint. A flat sacrum or a prominent sacrococcygeal joint will reduce the posterior sagittal diameter at this plane, and serious dystocia can occur in the second stage with failure in internal rotation.

The subpubic arch also compensates for the posterior sagittal diameter. The inter-ischial tuberosity diameter is a surrogate marker of subpubic angle. The subpubic angle should be more than 85°.

BASIC TYPES OF PELVIS

As mentioned in Chapter 1, there are four basic types of the pelvis (Figure 2.3a–d).

The gynecoid pelvis: The majority of women have this type of pelvis. The inlet is rounded, with the transverse diameter slightly bigger and slightly posteriorly set than the anteroposterior diameter. This is facilitated by the fact that the sacrum has a deep curve with an average inclination. This also ensures that the sacrosciatic notch is wide and shallow. The subpubic angle is obtuse. The sidewalls are parallel. Therefore, this type of pelvis has a good inter-ischial spine diameter and a good posterior sagittal diameter at all planes. This is conducive for engagement of a well-flexed occipito-anterior or transverse vertex in the pelvis and ensures the smooth progress of labour and birth (Figure 2.3a).

The android pelvis: In this type of pelvis, the inlet has a heart shape with beaking near the fore pelvis. The sacrum is stout and inclined forwards, resulting in shortening of the posterior sagittal diameters at the inlet. The sacrosciatic notch is narrow and deep. The side walls converge. This results in a uniform reduction of posterior sagittal diameter at all planes and a serious reduction of the transverse diameter at the plane of least pelvic dimensions. The compensatory subpubic angle is also acute and narrow and wastes a lot of space under the pubic symphysis. Therefore, there can be serious dystocia at all levels in this type of pelvis, more so at the level of ischial spines, i.e. obstetric

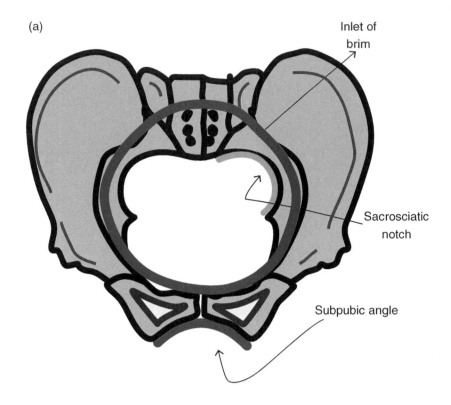

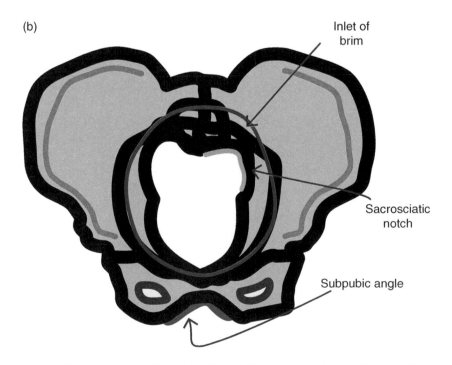

FIGURE 2.3   (a–d) The four types of the pelvis. The red line shows the shape of the inlet. The blue line the subpubic angle, and the green line the sacrosciatic notch.

(*Continued*)

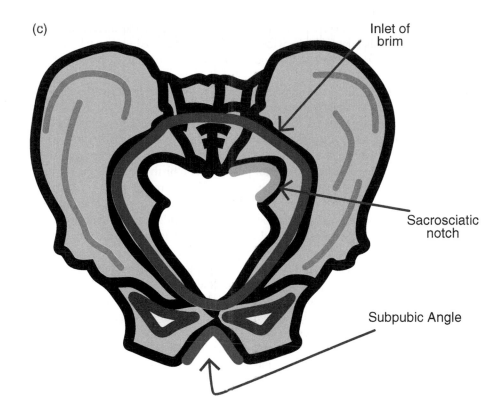

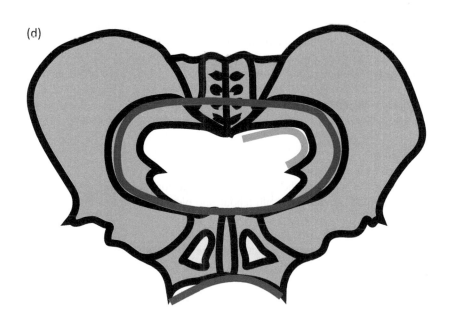

FIGURE 2.3 (*CONTINUED*)   (a–d) The four types of the pelvis. The red line shows the shape of the inlet. The blue line the subpubic angle, and the green line the sacrosciatic notch.

outlet, resulting in mid pelvic contraction and arrest in labour in the second stage. Since the anterior space under pubic symphysis is wasted, the widest diameter of the head is near the perineum. Any attempts at assisted delivery can cause serious perineal tears and, of course, birth asphyxia to the neonate (Figure 2.3c).

Anthropoid pelvis: Here, the inlet is an anteroposterior oval. At the inlet, the anteroposterior diameter is the largest. The sacrum is deep and inclined backwards. The side walls are parallel, and the sacrosciatic notches are wide but deep. The subpubic angle is obtuse, though lesser than the gynaecoid pelvis. The head more often uses the anteroposterior or oblique diameter of the inlet to engage. It is more likely to be occipito posterior. The internal rotation of the head is more likely to be posterior, resulting in a direct occipitoposterior position. The birth occurs as face to pubis delivery and is attended with a higher likelihood of perineal tears (Figure 2.3b).

Platypelloid pelvis: In this type of pelvis, the inlet is a transverse oval. The head invariably engages in the transverse diameter. There may be marked asynclitism as the anteroposterior diameter of the inlet is reduced. Sometimes the head may use only one half of the pelvis to engage if the anteroposterior diameter is too short. The fore pelvis and the subpubic angle, on the other hand, are wide and obtuse. The sacrum is more likely to be straight and with a prominent sacrococcygeal junction that could compromise the posterior sagittal diameter at the plane of least pelvis dimensions. The sacrosciatic notch is likely to be short and shallow. There can be serious dystocia at the level of the inlet of the pelvis and more likely to result in a delay in the engagement even in labour and cord prolapse even with vertex presentation.

The pelvis may not always be one in its type. It may be platypelloid in the upper strait and become gynaecoid in the lower strait. So the upper strait determines the parent type, and the terminology used for the lower strait is "tendency", in case if it is not the parent type. For example, we may have an anthropoid with an android tendency or a platypelloid with a gynaecoid tendency.

CLINICAL PELVIMETRY

It is a very important tool to assess the architecture of the pelvis. X-ray imaging is no longer done for pelvic assessment in the modern era to avoid radiation exposure to the fetus. Magnetic resonance imaging can be done to measure the diameters. MRI is also expensive and so has not found its use in day-to-day practice. Also, one must remember that the pelvis diameters can increase due to softening of maternal tissue and the backward movement of the coccyx. Further more, labour-induced moulding can help the fetus negotiate the pelvis.

Clinical internal pelvimetry, also called pelvic assessment, should be done near term or early labour.

A screen for pelvic adequacy in the antenatal clinic a week or so before the expected date of delivery should be performed. As a policy, we do a pelvic assessment at 38 weeks for

- All primigravida.
- All women with previous caesarean section.
- Multigravida with a big baby, short stature, or a posterior position.
- All women who had previous difficult labour and birth asphyxia or difficult instrumental delivery.

The clinical internal pelvimetry should be done after the woman has emptied her bowel and bladder.

Steps for Clinical Pelvimetry

Abdominal examination should be done before the pelvic assessment to note down the attitude of the head and position of the vertex. The women should be informed about the examination, its need, and the likely discomfort. This will help gain her cooperation.

The examination is done in a dorsal lithotomy position after taking all aseptic precautions.

Under aseptic precautions, the index and middle finger of the gloved right hand are introduced in the vagina as gently as possible. The cervix's status, consistency, effacement, and dilation of the cervix are noted. If the os admits a finger, then the membranes' status and the confirmation of the presenting part can also be done.

In a semi-pronated hand, an attempt is made with the tip of the middle finger to feel the sacral promontory. If it is felt, then a mark should be made on the hand at the level of the lower border of the pubic symphysis. Once the examination is completed and when the fingers are removed, it should be measured as the diagonal conjugate (Figure 2.4a). The hand is turned to pronation. The fingers should note down the curve of the sacrum from above downwards and from side to side. Any deviation from normal like flattening or straightening or prominence should be made a note of. The next focus is on the ischial spines. One should note down any prominence of the same. The inter-ischial spine distance should be measured with the pronated hand with the index finger on the right spine (Figure 2.4b). If the middle finger easily touches the left spine at the same time, then it is a matter of concern at the mid pelvis.

The next focus should be on the sacrosciatic notch. The sacrosciatic ligament should readily admit two fingers. Any deviation like a narrow or a high-arched sacrosciatic notch would mean a reduced distance between the ischial spine and the sacrum (posterior sagittal diameter). The side walls in front and above the ischial spine are palpated and observed for any convergence. The posterior sagittal diameter (PSD) at the plane of the least pelvic dimensions is the distance from the midpoint on inter-ischial spine line to the tip of the sacrum behind. If the ischial spine is closer to the sacrum, then this PSD reduces. This is reflected by the fact that the sacrosciatic notch becomes narrower, admitting less than two fingers. If the sacrococcygeal joint is jutting forward, it will also reduce the PSD.

The anterior-posterior diameter of the anatomical outlet extends from the lower border of the pubic symphysis to the tip of the coccyx. As the coccyx can move at the sacrococcygeal joint, it is likely to be pushed backwards by the advancing head in labour, thereby further increasing the anteroposterior diameter. The subpubic angle is measured by direct palpation by approximating the middle and index finger of the pronated hand inside the vagina under the pubic arch. The two fingers should be easily fit under the pubic arch (Figure 2.4c). Alternately, we can place the index and the middle finger of the left hand over the two inferior rami from above standing on the right side of the woman and observe the angle between the two fingers. Ideally, the angle should be obtuse. The depth or thickness, the height, and the angle of inclination of the pubic symphysis should also be noted. The pubis symphysis should have a forward inclination and should not be very wide or long.

The transverse diameter of the anatomical outlet is assessed after the fingers are withdrawn from the vagina. The narrowest diameter is the transverse diameter. The transverse diameter is measured by inserting the knuckle of the fisted right hand in pronation between the two ischial tuberosities (Figure 2.4d). This can be performed when the tuberosities are freed. So, the woman should assume a lithotomy position or hyperflex her thighs towards the abdomen in a dorsal lithotomy position. The four knuckles should comfortably fit between the two tuberosities for the diameter to be considered adequate. Before withdrawing the fingers out, we can take an opportunity to sweep and stretch the membranes around the internal os in an attempt to encourage the spontaneous onset of labour.

When a particular diameter is suspected to be borderline, a special note should be made of the compensatory diameter (described above).

External Pelvimetry

These are measurements taken externally to predict the possibility of problems in the pelvis.

These are estimated with the help of external callipers. This is detailed in Chapter 12.

(a)

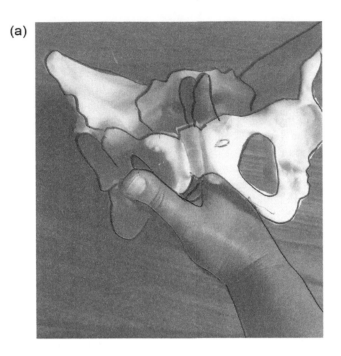

(b)

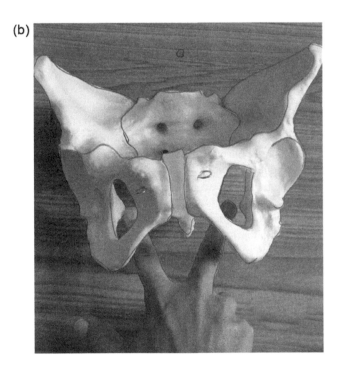

FIGURE 2.4 (a–d) The pelvic assessment concept on the pelvis.

(Continued)

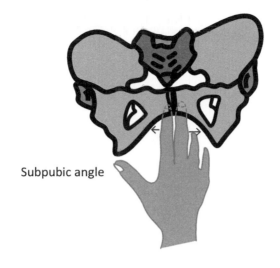

Subpubic angle

(d)

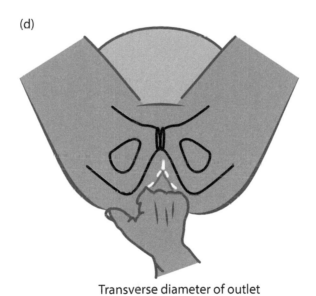

Transverse diameter of outlet
with the knuckles of the hand

FIGURE 2.4 (*CONTINUED*) (a–d) The pelvic assessment concept on the pelvis.

SUGGESTED READING

Siccardi MA, Imonugo O, Valle C. *Anatomy, abdomen and pelvis, pelvic inlet.* (updated 2021 Mar 16) In StatPearls [Internet]. Treasure Island (FL): StarPearl's publishing; 2021 Jan, Available at https://www.ncbi.nlm.nih.gov › books › NBK519068.

3 Understanding the Passenger

Gowri Dorairajan
Jawaharlal Institute of Postgraduate Medical
Education and Research (JIPMER)

In normal labour, the fetus presents as the vertex. The head of the fetus is the most incompressible part. It is important to understand the static and dynamic diameter of the fetal skull. The static ones are fixed. The dynamic diameters change depending on the attitude of the head. Let us understand the fetal skull. It is made up of many bones. The base of the skull is ossified and united at birth and cannot be easily compressed, whereas the cranium can undergo compression. The cranial bones are weakly ossified thin and compressible at birth. The cranial bones are separated by membranous gaps called sutures, giving a possibility of overlap during labour.

The head has two ovoids: the transverse and the longitudinal. The transverse ovoid is widest at the parietal eminence level and has fixed static diameters.

The longitudinal ovoid is dynamic, and the dimensions can change depending on the degree of flexion or deflection.

The fetal skull has three parts: the vault of the cranium, the base, and the face, including the jaw.

FOCUSING ON THE VAULT

The cranium or vault has two parietal bones on each side — one occipital bone posteriorly and two frontal bones in the front (Figure 3.1a). These bones are separated by sutures that are nothing but membranous space. Identifying the sutures during vaginal examination are key findings to determine the position of the head. There are four sutures: the coronal suture between the frontal bones and the two parietal bones, the sagittal suture between the two parietal bones, and the lambdoid suture that separates the occipital bone from the parietal bones. The frontal suture between the two frontal bones extends from the glabella to the anterior end of the bregma.

Fontanelles: The meeting place of the four bones in front and the three bones behind is separated by a space called fontanella.

Anterior fontanella or bregma: This is a diamond-shaped membranous space at the junction of the two frontal bones in the front and the two parietal bones behind and on the sides. This is a membranous depression with one suture radiating out of all the four corners of the diamond: the frontal suture in front of the coronal sutures on the sides and the sagittal suture behind. The bregma itself measures 3×2 cm, and it gets ossified at 1.5 years of age.

THE CLINICAL SIGNIFICANCE OF BREGMA

- Palpation of Bregma at vaginal examination during labour signifies a deflexed head. It is usually not palpable on vaginal examination.
- Reflects the intracranial pressure as bulging membranes when high and depressed membrane when low.
- It helps in accommodating the growing brain inside the skull, given the skull base is ossified and not likely to expand.

The posterior fontanelle or lambda is felt as a bony depression and marks the meeting point of the sagittal and the lambdoid suture. It is felt as a Y-shaped depression without any membrane separation. It ossifies by 1.5 to 2 months of life.

DOI: 10.1201/9781003034360-3

IMPORTANT LANDMARKS

Occiput: The protuberance on the occipital bone is an important landmark. It is the denominator or the reference point for vertex presentation (Figure 3.1b).

Vertex*:* It is a rectangular area bounded anteriorly by the coronal suture, posteriorly by the lambdoid suture, and on both sides by an imaginary line from the parietal eminences.

Glabella: The area between the orbital ridges.

Nasion: The root of the nose.

Sinciput*:* The bony prominence between the glabella below and the anterior limit of bregma above (prominence of the forehead)

Sub-occiput: The junction of the neck and the occiput. This is just below the prominence of the occiput.

Mentum: The midpoint on the chin (jaw bone).

Sub-mentum: Is the junction of the neck with the chin (the point just below the chin).

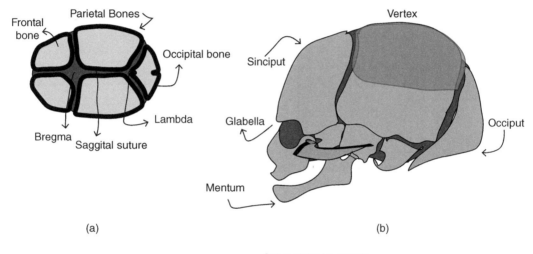

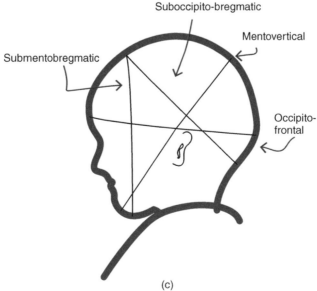

FIGURE 3.1   (a) Vault of the head. (b) Lateral view with landmarks. (c) Diameters of the head.

Brow: Is an area bounded by the anterior end of the bregma and the coronal suture on one side and by the nasion and the supraorbital ridges on the other side.

Face: Extends from the nasion and the supraorbital ridges above to the junction of the floor of the mouth and the neck below.

DIAMETERS OF THE FETAL SKULL

The static diameters: The transverse diameters are static. However, they can change in labour due to overlapping (moulding).

- **Biparietal diameter**: It extends between the two parietal eminences. It is the broadest and measures 9.5 cm. It is set a little posteriorly from the mid coronal plane of the body.
- **Bitemporal diameter**: Extends between the two temporal bones. It measures about 8 cm.
- **Bimastoid diameter**: Extends between the two mastoid bones and measures 7.5 cm.
- **Super-sub parietal diameter**: From a point below the parietal eminence to a point just above the parietal eminence of the opposite side. It is 8.5 cm, and the fetus engages with this diameter instead of the biparietal diameter to negotiate a flat pelvis.

The dynamic longitudinal diameters (Figure 3.1c): The longitudinal diameter changes depending on the degree of deflexion and extension (attitude) of the head.
Diameters of vertex presentation:

- **Suboccipito-bregmatic diameter**: This extends from the suboccipital (just below the occipital prominence) to the centre of the bregma. It measures 9.5 cm. This is the diameter of engagement of the fetal skull in a well-flexed vertex presentation.
- **Suboccipito-frontal diameter**: Extends from the sub-occiput to the anterior end of the bregma. It is about 10 cm. It presents mild deflexion of the head.
- **Occipito-frontal**: This longitudinal diameter of the fetal head in a moderately deflexed head extends from the occipital protuberance to the glabella and measures about 11.5 cm.

Deflexed heads at the onset of labour are seen in occipito-posterior positions.

- **Diameters of extended head**: If instead of flexion, the head is in an attitude of extension, then the following diameters of the fetus engage in the pelvis.
- **Submentobregmatic**: Is seen in the completely extended head resulting in face presentation. It extends from just below the chin to the centre of the bregma. This also measures around 9.5 cm.
- **Submentovertical**: The longitudinal diameter when the extension is incomplete. It extends from below the chin to the highest point on the sagittal suture (just in front of the posterior fontanelle). It measures 11.5 cm.
- **Mentovertical**: The diameter of engagement in case of brow presentation (incompletely extended head). It extends from the chin to the highest point on the sagittal suture (in front of the lambda). It is the longest diameter, measuring 13.5 cm. The labour will come to a standstill in brow presentation unless the head completely extends to the face or flexes to become vertex.

SUMMARY OF THE DIAMETERS OF ENGAGEMENT OF THE FETUS

The definition of engagement refers to the biparietal diameter crossing the pelvic brim. This transverse diameter of the fetal skull is constant for all. The longitudinal diameters used by the fetal head while engaging change depending on the head's attitude. Hence, this dynamic diameter is the reference diameter of engagement of the fetal skull.

- Vertex fully flexed head: Suboccipito-bregmatic diameter.
- Vertex deflexed head: Suboccipito-frontal (occipito-posterior position).
- Vertex moderately deflexed: Occipito-frontal (occipito-posterior position).
- Brow (incompletely extended head): Mentovertical.
- Face (completely extended) : Submentobregmatic.

The circumference of the fetal skull in a well-flexed head at the suboccipito-bregmatic plane is about 33 cm, and it increases by a centimetre in the occipito-frontal plane.

Therefore, a well-flexed head ensures the smallest ovoid leads the fetus in labour.

4 Stages of Labour

Gowri Dorairajan
Jawaharlal Institute of Postgraduate Medical
Education and Research (JIPMER)

Definition of normal labour: Labour refers to the various events and changes that occur in the reproductive tract and maternal pelvis during the process of bringing forth the fetus into the world, that is, during the natural process of childbirth. The following clause is an important part of the definition of normal labour.

Normal labour refers to a spontaneous onset, at term, in a singleton fetus presenting as vertex that completes spontaneously, resulting in vaginal delivery without any aid or complications.

So actually, normal labour is a retrospective diagnosis. The hallmark of labour is the onset of the painful uterine contraction and ends with the birth of the fetus and the placenta. Normal labour involves a lot of changes in the reproductive tract and adaptive movements by the descending fetus to complete its journey through the pelvis successfully.

Stages of labour: Normal labour is divided into **four stages**.

First stage: This is characterized by the onset of painful uterine contractions. The goal is to achieve complete opening of the cervical canal from a closed organ to 10 cm dilation (full dilation) to let the fetus (engaging with a longitudinal suboccipito-bregmatic diameter of 9.5 cm and transverse biparietal diameter of 9.5 cm) pass through it comfortably. So, the stage of labour till the cervix dilates fully is the first stage of labour.

Second stage: Refers to the phase from full dilation of the cervix till the birth of the fetus to the outside world.

Third stage: Refers to the expulsion of the placenta and the membrane.

Fourth stage: Defined by some to include the first hour after delivery of the placenta. The first hour being the most crucial for the occurrence of any complications; the woman should be closely observed during this stage.

Let us understand the events during each stage in detail.

FIRST STAGE OF LABOUR

This phase is from the onset of uterine contractions till full dilation of the cervix.

It is the most extended phase of labour.

Duration: It lasts for a variable period of 8–18 hours in a primigravid and 4–10 hours in a multigravida.

The contractions are intermittent and painful and become more frequent and vigorous as labour advances.

EVENTS DURING THE FIRST STAGE

Dilatation and effacement of the cervix

Normally the cervix hangs inside the vagina as a 3- to 5-cm long organ. During the first stage of labour, the cervix gets taken up with the uterus and loses its distinction as a separate hanging organ. This is called effacement (Figure 4.1a and c).

DOI: 10.1201/9781003034360-4

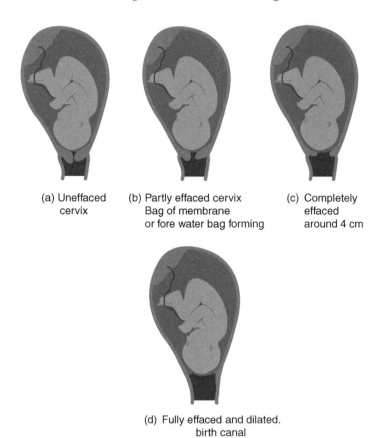

(a) Uneffaced cervix

(b) Partly effaced cervix Bag of membrane or fore water bag forming

(c) Completely effaced around 4 cm

(d) Fully effaced and dilated. birth canal

FIGURE 4.1 Cervical dilation and effacement, a bag of membrane, and formation of the birth canal. Pink colour represents the cervix, red the uterus, brown the vagina and green the amniotic membrane.

The external os opens up slowly to 10 cm dilation.

Mechanism: The upper part of the uterus has an abundance of longitudinal muscle fibres, whereas the lower part, including the cervix, has more circular fibres. The most important character of uterine muscle contraction of the upper part of the uterus is retraction, which means shortening of the myofibril after each contraction. When the longitudinal muscle fibre attached to circular fibre shortens, the circular fibre is bound to get taken up and open or dilate.

Formation of the bag of membranes: The fetus is in a sac with an amnion towards the fetus and the chorion towards the uterus. With the onset of contractions and opening of the cervix, the membranes separate from the lower part of the fetus close to the internal os. With increased intrauterine pressure, this fore membrane bulges with amniotic fluid proximal to the advancing head. This is called the formation of the bag of membranes. In occipito-anterior position, this bag of the membrane is spherical or watch glass type and bulges evenly every time the intrauterine pressure rises during uterine contraction. This bulging membrane acts as an important dilator of the cervix (Figure 4.1b).

Fetal axis pressure: Normally, the fetal axis through the spine coincides with the longitudinal axis of the uterus. During labour, the fetus aligns itself so that the contraction force passing through the fetal spine pushes it along the curve of Carus. The well-fitting descending head stretches and thrusts itself over the os of the cervix and, along with the uterine force propelling it downwards, acts as a cervical dilator. *The shortening myofibril* of the upper segment gives an upward pull. These three working in synchrony bring about the dilation of the cervix. The absence of this alignment and emptiness of the lower segment in the transverse lie brings out the reason why the cervix appears like a hanging loose, thick, and incompletely dilated organ. This also explains the delay in dilation when the presenting part is ill-fitting, like the footling breech, or when the fetus is misaligned due to the pendulous abdomen.

It is important to understand the difference in the first stage of labour in a multi- and primigravida. In a primigravid woman, effacement precedes dilation, whereas, in a multigravida, the dilation starts first. So a fully effaced 1-cm dilated cervix for a primigravida is a favourable finding. A multigravida is more likely to have a finding of 2-cm dilation with an uneffaced cervix. In a good proportion of primigravida, the effacement starts in the last trimester even before painful contractions set in.

THE PHASES OF THE FIRST STAGE OF LABOUR

From the onset of uterine contractions to the full dilatation of the cervix, the first stage goes through various phases. The duration of each phase is variable.

Latent phase: This is a phase where the uterine contractions are palpable, and the woman experiences some form of pain, but the cervical changes are none or slow and gradual.

This phase is longer in those who did not have a mature cervix before the onset of labour and those where labour is induced. In this phase, the cervix softens and becomes more pliable. The contractions become more regular and coordinated. Some women may get exhausted in the latent phase itself. Propagation beyond the cut-off limits forewarns about difficult active phase and cephalopelvic disproportion.

Active phase: This is a phase marked by steady dilation of the cervix with more frequent regular and intensified uterine contractions. The cervix dilates at least by 1 cm every hour. It may proceed at a faster rate of 1.5–2 cm/hour in a multigravida. The definition of the active phase has changed over the years. From 3 cm in the late 1990s to 4 cm since 2008, the recent recommendation by the WHO is that the active phase starts when the cervix is 5 cm dilated. The dilation of the cervix proceeds linearly (1 cm/hour after the active phase), as depicted in the partograph. This is an important landmark to anticipate the time of delivery and start charting the progress in a partogram.

Because of rising caesarean section rates with half-hearted attempts at vaginal delivery and cervical dystocia documented as an indication for labour, the Consortium of Labour has recently revised the designation of active phase when the cervix is 6 cm instead of 4 cm dilated

This revised definition has to be interpreted with caution in cases of a trial of labour in cephalopelvic disproportion and the presence of overt features of cephalopelvic disproportion.

The active phase has an initial *phase of acceleration followed by a phase of maximum slope*. During this phase, the dilation of the cervix proceeds linearly (1 cm or more per hour).

This is followed by a deceleration phase (also called a transition phase) where the dilation becomes tardy. Maximum descent occurs in this phase. The prolonged deceleration phase of the active part of labour alerts about likely problems of labour related to descent and rotation of the head (Figure 4.2).

Descent of head: The descent of the head also varies over time, even in active labour. During the phase of maximum slope and transition phase, maximum descent of the head occurs, achieving 1 cm/hour and up to 2 cm/hour in the transition phase. The distance from the sacral promontory to the tip of the coccyx is 9–10 cm. This is the distance the fetus has to travel from the brim till it is born. Therefore, marking the descent in centimetres in the partogram is more aptly representative of the descent of the fetal head. The head may be at lower stations in a primigravida in early labour compared to a multigravida. The head is likely to be above the brim at the onset of labour in a multigravida. There may be only minimal descent in early labour and maximum descent in the transition and second stages of labour.

EVENTS IN THE SECOND STAGE OF LABOUR

The second stage of labour starts from full dilation of the cervix till the expulsion of the fetus to the outside world. Substantial descent occurs in this stage of labour.

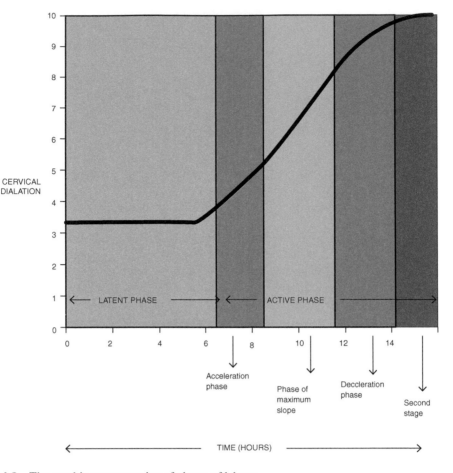

FIGURE 4.2   The graphic representation of phases of labour.

The bag of membrane invariably ruptures if it is still intact.

The uterine contractions become stronger and more frequent and may last up to 60 seconds. With the fetal axis aligning with the uterine axis, each contraction and retraction of the myofibril propels the fetus downwards to the pelvic floor. This is the propulsive phase of the second stage. This phase is *passive* at the beginning. The retraction of uterine myofibril after every contraction is an important property in achieving the expulsion of the fetus from the cervical canal to the lower vagina. The tug of the retraction power works over the cervix fixed with the help of the triradiate ligament.

Once the head reaches lower down to the pelvic floor and distends the lower vagina, the woman gets an urge to push (*active phase*). The voluntary expulsive forces aid the uterine propulsive force in achieving the birth of the fetus. In between the contractions, the head tends to recoil up due to the elasticity of the tissues. Though the head seems to recoil back, there is a steady descent of the head. When it reaches and stretches the perineum and the vaginal outlet, it no longer recoils back (crowning), and maternal active pushing (bearing down) successfully delivers the fetus.

Formation of birth canal: With progressively intensifying uterine contractions., the cervix gets completely taken up (effaced or merges with the uterine wall). The cervix cannot be differentiated from the uterine wall as a separate organ projecting in the vagina. When the cervix dilates fully, it merges with the vagina, and the fornices disappear. So in the second stage, the uterus, cervix, and vagina become one canal or a single conduit without an individual identity (Figure 4.1d). This is called the birth canal. This concept helps to understand the problems that can happen while doing a caesarean section in the second stage of labour.

EVENTS IN THE THIRD STAGE OF LABOUR

This stage starts after the birth of the fetus and completes after the expulsion of the placenta. The placenta, which is a discoid structure spanning nearly 15–20 cm in diameter, occupies almost one-third of the uterine wall at term. It has 8–10 cotyledons on the maternal surface and weighs around 500 gm. The membranes cover the fetal side, and usually, the cord is attached in the centre.

Once the fetus is born, there is a sudden decrease in the surface area of the uterus. This shears the placental attachment site and initiates the separation of the placenta, aided by yet another strong contraction and retraction of the uterus. Finally, there is venous occlusion and rupture of the vessels underlying the placenta.

The separation can begin from the margin of the placenta (*marginal or Mathew Duncan method*) of separation or start in the centre of the placenta and proceed to the margins (*Schultze's method of separation*). The separation results in blood accumulating behind the placenta from the exposed spiral arterioles that slowly spread to the placenta's entire undersurface, resulting in the complete separation and detachment of the decidual plate from the basal layer of the decidua. Once completely separated, the placenta is ready to be expelled (Figure 4.3a and b).

After the placenta is expelled, the firmly contracted and retracted uterus squeezes close to the spiral vessels running across the uterine wall. This firm contraction and retraction are essential to arrest the bleeding after delivery of the fetus and the placenta.

Signs of placental separation: The following are the signs of placental separation in the order of occurrence.

The reappearance of uterine contractions is the starting point to further initiate the placental attachment.

This is followed by a gush of bleed from the placenta's undersurface, as mentioned above.

True lengthening of the cord occurs when the placenta gets detached and comes to the lower part of the uterus. The cord outside the vagina starts lengthening.

Suprapubic bulge means the detached placenta gets pushed to the lower segment and fills the lower segment.

DURATION OF THE STAGES OF LABOUR

It is an adage that no woman should see the sunrise or sunset twice in labour. This means that the labour should not last longer than 24 hours. Therefore, we should be aware of the average time spent in each of these stages of labour. The time depends on the parity as also as the type of labour.

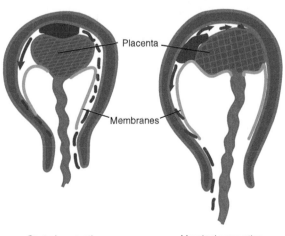

FIGURE 4.3   Figure depicting the placental separation.

Labour is likely to be longer in induced labour, especially when the cervix was not very ripe to begin with. Detailed below is the time spent in the various stages.

Latent phase: It may last on an average of 8–10 hours. More often, the woman may present in active labour directly. The upper limit for an optimal outcome is not more than 20 hours in a primigravida and 14 hours in a multigravida.

The first stage of labour: This average lasts from 10 to 12 hour duration in a primigravida and 6–8 hours in a multigravida woman. Once active labour of 4 cm dilation is reached, the first stage would take about 4–6 hours.

The second stage of labour: Typically, a primigravida may take 1 hour to sometimes up to 2 hours. With regional analgesia, the second stage may get extended to 3 hours. A multigravida would take 0.5 hours on average. The maximum time limit in a multigravida is 1 hour without and 2 hours with regional analgesia. The active bearing down phase in a primigravida should not be longer than 1 hour in a primigravida and half hour in a multigravida.

Third stage: This stage lasts for about 15 minutes to half an hour. Prolongation beyond 1 hour is of concern. In modern obstetrics, with the active management of the third stage of labour, the third stage may last from 5 to 15 minutes only.

The following factors affect the duration of labour

1. **Type of onset of labour**: Induced labour is likely to be longer than spontaneous onset.
2. **Parity**: As already discussed, primigravida takes longer than multigravida.
3. **Position of the head**: Occipito-posterior positions of the head take a longer time to complete the rotation.
4. A tense mind is a tense cervix is an adage. Therefore, a fearful, anxious woman would take longer to dilate the cervix.
5. Abruption and amnioinfusion can enhance labour by increasing intrauterine pressure.
6. Overdistension of the uterus due to multiple pregnancies or hydramnios can lengthen labour due to incoordinate uterine contractions.

Thus, the pelvis architecture, synchronized power of the uterus, the size of the fetus, the psyche of the mother, and the tissue resistance influence the duration of labour.

5 Understanding the Power
The Uterine Contractions

Gowri Dorairajan
Jawaharlal Institute of Postgraduate Medical
Education and Research (JIPMER)

Uterine contraction is the hallmark of labour. The contractions progressively increase in intensity, frequency, and duration to achieve the goal of full dilation and descent of the fetus to achieve successful vaginal birth of the fetus.

NORMAL UTERINE CONTRACTIONS

a. **Pacemakers**: The pacemakers for the contractions are near the ostia at the fundus of the uterus. The contraction initiated at the ostia spreads all around the uterus and spreads downwards towards the lower segment with a lag of about 10 seconds. There is perfect synchrony in the occurrence of the contractions from both the ostial ends (Figure 11.1a).

b. **Polarity**: The normal uterine contractions are such that there is fundal dominance. The contractions start from the pacemaker and spread all around as well as to the lower part of the uterus. The lowermost part, called the lower segment, remains passive and only dilates and stretches. The cervix has circular fibres that attach to the longitudinal muscle fibres of the upper segment.

c. **Retraction**: Retraction of the uterine myofibril is an important and unique feature of the uterine muscle. After every contraction, there is a slight reduction in the size of the myofibril. This property is called retraction. It means the uterine myofibrils do not return to the original length after a contraction. The retraction helps dilation by tugging the cervix open while the contraction helps in the propulsion of the fetus. This can be likened to the cover of a bolster purse stringed at one end. If we want to remove the bolster from the cover, the purse string is opened. The thumbs push the bolster while the fingers shorten the length of the cover by frilling it. The longitudinal fibres of the upper segment are like the bolster cover and must retract and shorten. The round head, similar to the smooth leading portion of the bolster, acts as a dilator. The circular fibres of the cervix are similar to the purse string end and open passively.

d. The uterine contractions have the following features.

Intensity: The rise in intrauterine pressure with each contraction signifies the intensity. The intensity goes on increasing to achieve a pressure of up to 80–100 mm of mercury. It is clinically perceived as the hardness and inability to indent the uterus at the peak of contraction denotes good intensity. It is objectively measured in *Montevideo units*. The intrauterine pressure generated with every contraction in a 10 minute window is added to arrive at the Montevideo units. Montevideo units of 180–200 are considered good contractions to ensure good progress of labour.

Contractions are perceived as pain because the raised intrauterine pressure causes the transient hypoxia of the smooth muscles. Pain also occurs due to stretching of the overlying peritoneum. The dilation of the cervix and stretching of the nerve roots also contribute to pain. Finally, at the second stage, the advancing head on the perineum causes somatic pain.

DOI: 10.1201/9781003034360-5

Tone: This represents the basal intrauterine pressure in between the contractions. The uterus must relax completely in between contractions to allow good oxygenation to the fetus. The basal tone is less than 8–12 mm of mercury.

The intrauterine pressure is governed by the uterine muscle contractility and the contents of the uterus (multiple gestations). Polyhydramnios and concealed abruption can increase the pressure.

Duration: The time for which a contraction lasts may vary from 10 to 15 seconds in early labour to up to 40–45 seconds late in labour. The duration may extend to 45–60 seconds during the second stage of labour.

Frequency: The contraction in early labour may be as infrequent as once in 15–20 minutes. They progressively become frequent and occur every 2.5 to 3 minutes. The uterine contractions should not exceed more than five in 10 minutes. Too frequent contractions are not good as they will exhaust the mother and compromise fetal oxygenation.

Synchrony and coordination: The contractions starting near the ostia propagate to the rest of the uterus with great coordination. They reach the lower part of the uterus a few seconds later but reach the highest intensity faster than the upper segment. Thus, the duration of the contraction also keeps waning from the fundus to the lower part of the uterus. The intensity also reduces as it reaches the lower segment from the fundus of the uterus. Thus, the coordinated contractions ensure that the whole uterus contracts at the same time at the peak of a contraction, with the upper segment being most intense. The lag in duration and intensity ensures the whole uterus relaxes at the same time.

Optimum contraction lasts for 40 seconds and raises the uterine pressure by 60–80 mm of Hg, and recurs every 2.5 to 3 minutes.

Biomolecular basis of uterine contraction: The uterine myofibril has actin and myosin proteins. The former produces thin and the latter dense contractile filaments – the two crosslink to bring about the contraction. The myosin protein has to be activated by phosphorylation. This activation is brought out by light-chain kinase in the presence of the calmodulin calcium complex. Any stimulus that increases intracellular calcium level will increase the contraction. Calcium concentration increases when oxytocin receptors bind oxytocin. This is brought out by stimulating phospholipase C and cyclic adenosine monophosphate (cAMP), which help release calcium from the sarcoplasmic reticulum. Prostaglandins stimulate calcium release. Progesterone and alpha-adrenergic increase while beta-adrenergic reduces cAMP, and hence the intracellular calcium levels.

Measurement of Uterine Activity

The uterine activity can be measured by objective means and or subjective assessment. Uterine contractions can be objectively measured with

a. External tocodynamometer
b. Internal intrauterine pressure monitor
c. Electromyography

External tocodynamometer: This measures the pressure exerted by a transducer with a mechanical piston that raises as the contraction starts. The drawback is that the measurements are subject to variations in maternal posture, tightness of strapping the transducer to the abdomen, and it can get affected by the maternal rise of intra-abdominal pressure. The measurements include frequency of contractions, peak to peak time, and fall-to-rise ratio (time from peak to fall of pressure to baseline divided by the time from start to end of the rise in pressure). It helps determine the frequency, duration, and resting time between contractions. It can give a moderate assessment of the timing of the decelerations. The advantage is that it is non-invasive and yet objective to a certain extent. The normal contraction curve is bell shaped for it to be effective. If the time taken for the contraction to fall is more than the time taken to rise, then it causes uterine muscle fatigue, and the contractions may not be effective enough. High fall-to-rise ratios during labour are associated with a higher risk of caesarean section [1].

Internal uterine pressure: This is carried out by a pressure measuring catheter inserted into the uterine cavity. It requires rupturing of the membranes and is invasive. This method is a fairly accurate method to measure the pressure generated during contractions. It helps in determining the frequency, duration, resting pressure, and pressure generated with uterine contractions. The pressure is expressed as *Montevideo units*. This was developed by Caldeyro-Barcia in 1969. It is the sum of the rise (peak minus baseline pressure) in uterine pressure caused by all the contractions in a 10-minute window. *Alexandria unit* is another method of expressing uterine contractions. It is obtained by multiplying the Montevideo unit with the average duration of contractions in 10 minutes. Two hundred Montevideo units are considered optimal and adequate for bringing about the progress of dilation of the cervix and descent of the head. The optimal uterine contraction needed to complete labour also depends on the tissue resistance to be overcome. Measuring these units has been recommended to predict labour dystocia and improve an evidence-based approach for dystocia in labour [2].

Electromyography: This is achieved with electrodes placed at various places over the abdomen to note the activity from the underlying uterine contractions. The power density, spatiotemporal mapping, and entropy can be studied. This method, however, cannot measure the amplitude. It can measure the frequency, duration, polarity, and uterine fatigue due to overactivity. It can also measure the coordination of the uterine activity and help in the prediction of dystocia [1].

FORMATION OF THE UTERINE SEGMENTS

During the latter half of pregnancy, the lower segment starts forming. During labour, the uterus gets delineated into an actively contracting upper segment and a passively dilating and stretching lower segment.

LOWER SEGMENT

This part is derived from the isthmus of the uterus. Isthmus is an area between the anatomical and the histological internal os (the latter is distal to the former). In the nonpregnant state, it measures around 1 mm. At the peak of labour and in the second stage, the lower segment extends from 5 to 7 cm. The lower segment starts forming in the late third trimester (after 34–36 weeks) and is most well-formed in late labour.

The lower segment and the cervix have more circular fibres, which attach the stronger longitudinal fibres of the upper segment. The duration of uterine contractions diminishes from the fundus to the lower segment. The contractions generated near the fundus reach the lower segment after a lag of 10–20 seconds. So, the advanced contraction in the upper segment displaces the amniotic fluid downwards. This helps in forming a rounded bag of the membrane in front of the presenting part, which helps dilate the cervix passively.

Anatomical identification of the lower segment: It is that part of the uterus which lies under the loose utero-vesical fold of the peritoneum. This is an essential landmark while performing lower segment caesarean section. So, the round ligaments mark the upper limit of the lower segment on the sides.

Clinical importance of lower segment: The lower segment being passive is the area that should be incised while performing a caesarean section. The lower segment incisions remain undisturbed, unlike the upper segment, which undergoes contraction and retraction in the puerperium while the uterus undergoes involution. The thickness of the lower segment in labour varies from 2 to 5 mm. The lower segment may get extremely thinned out and stretched out in obstructed labour and may become papery thin, easily torn while doing caesarean for second stage arrest or obstructed labour.

Lower segment measurement by sonography is an important assessment for women with previous caesarean at term to determine the eligibility for vaginal delivery.

UPPER SEGMENT

The upper segment is the part of the uterus in labour that is above the level of the round ligaments. This is the most important active part of the uterus during labour. The myofibers actively contract and retract during labour. The upper segment is thicker, with many blood-filled sinuses running across the muscles. Therefore, incisions in the upper segment tend to form micro-hematomas. The incision line gets constantly disturbed after delivery due to the retraction during involution. Therefore, upper segment incisions do not heal well and have a higher risk of rupture in subsequent pregnancy and labour. The upper segment feels like the well contracted firm uterus immediately after delivery.

REFERENCES

1. American College of Obstetricians and Gynecologists (College); Society for Maternal-Fetal Medicine; Caughey AB, Cahill AG, Guise JM, Rouse DJ. Safe prevention of the primary cesarean delivery. *Am J Obstet Gynecol*. 2014; 210(3): 179–193.
2. Kissler KJ, Lowe NK, Hernandez TL. An integrated review of uterine activity monitoring for evaluating labor dystocia. *J Midwifery Women's Health*. 2020; 65(3): 323–334. doi: 10.1111/jmwh.13119. Epub 2020 Jun 1. PMID: 32478978; PMCID: PMC7875314.

6 Understanding the Fetal Journey

Gowri Dorairajan
Jawaharlal Institute of Postgraduate Medical
Education and Research (JIPMER)

The goal of the fetal journey through the passage of the maternal pelvis is a successful vaginal delivery and to be born crying lusciously without asphyxia. The fetal journey is aided by the uterine contractions and the elastic recoil of the pelvic floor.

IMPORTANT DEFINITIONS AND TERMINOLOGIES

It is important to understand the following terminologies referred to often in labour.

1. **Lie**: It is the relation of the longitudinal axis of the fetus to the longitudinal axis of the uterus. The longitudinal axis of the fetus passes through the spine. When the spine is in line with the longitudinal axis of the uterus (line from the fundus to the lower segment), it is a longitudinal lie. When the fetal axis is perpendicular to the uterine axis, it is a transverse lie. When the fetal axis is at an angle to the uterine axis, it is an oblique lie (Figure 6.1a).
2. **Presentation**: This refers to the part of the fetus occupying the lower pole of the uterus. If the head is in the lower pole, it is a cephalic presentation, and when it is the podalic pole, it is called breech presentation. In a transverse lie, the shoulders occupy the lower pole, and hence it is referred to as shoulder presentation.
3. **Presenting part**: This refers to that part of the fetus which overlies the internal os and is thus going to be born first. The presenting part in a cephalic presentation can be either vertex or brow or face (Figure 6.1b). In breech, it can be buttocks and genitalia (extended breech or buttocks, genitalia, and feet (flexed breech), or only feet (footling breech)).
4. **Engagement**: When the biparietal diameter of the fetal skull crosses the pelvic brim, the head is said to be engaged. It is expected that the station can be "–1" or "0" when the head is engaged because the distance between the biparietal plane and the leading vertex is about 5 cm. Five centimetres is also the distance from the pelvic brim to the level of the ischial spines.
5. **Denominator**: It is a fixed reference bony point on the fetal skull for the given presenting part. This denominator is used as a reference to determine the position of the head to the maternal pelvis. The following is the list of denominators for the various presenting parts:

   - Vertex: occiput
   - Face: mentum
   - Brow: mentum
   - Breech: sacrum
   - Transverse lie: accromium

6. **Attitude**: It is the relationship of the various parts of the fetus to each other. There is normally flexion at every joint, including the atlantooccipital joint. This is called as attitude of universal flexion (Figure 6.1c). This is important to ensure the smallest ovoid longitudinally

DOI: 10.1201/9781003034360-6

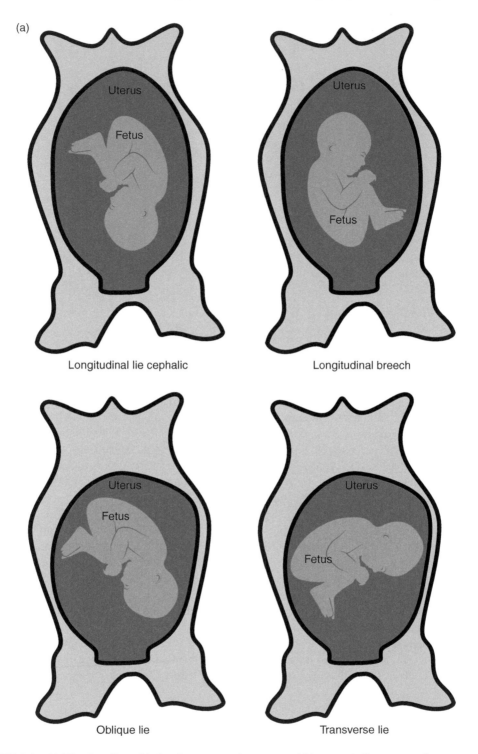

FIGURE 6.1 (a) The four lies; (b) the three presenting parts within a cephalic presentation; and (c) the universal flexion.

(Continued)

(b)

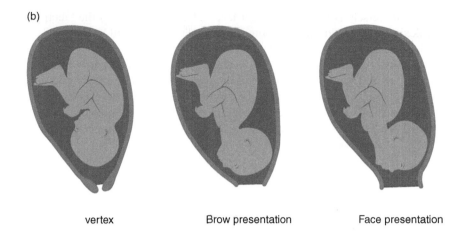

vertex   Brow presentation   Face presentation

(c)

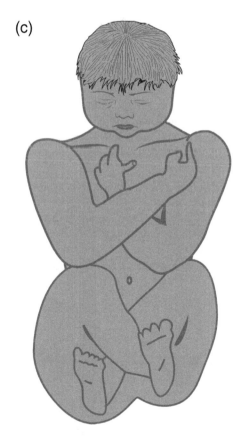

FIGURE 6.1 (*CONTINUED*)   (a) The four lies; (b) the three presenting parts within a cephalic presentation; and (c) the universal flexion.

as well as transversely at hip and shoulder levels. This is also called the "fetal position". Lack of flexion at the head can cause bigger diameters of the skull negotiating the pelvis and can be the source of trouble in some situations.

7. **Position**: Position is termed based on the relation of the denominator to the various quadrants of the pelvis. The position can be left or right, and it can be anterior, transverse, or posterior depending on the placement of the denominator in the concerned presenting part. So, for example, in vertex presentation, we can have left occipito-anterior (LOA) position, left occipito-transverse (LOT), and left occipito-posterior (LOP) positions and similar three on the right side (Figure 6.2).

UNDERSTANDING FETAL POSITION BY ABDOMINAL EXAMINATION

Abdominal examination forms a critical examination to assess the fetal position. One must carefully and mindfully note the fetal position and document it at the onset of labour. The findings may become more and more obscured due to contractions, decrease liquor, and engaged head as the labour advances. The initial notes would be of great relevance when the caput and moulding mask the findings on internal examination late in labour. Of course, intrapartum ultrasound might help know where the back is but thorough mindful examination at the beginning of labour is quite accurate and reliable.

Inspection of the abdomen gives a good idea about the overall volume occupied, the flattening below the umbilicus raising suspicion of occipito-posterior positions, the tone of the abdominal wall, the presence of pendulous abdomen, any scars on the abdomen, and oedema and obesity of the abdominal wall. Sub-umbilical flattening will be observed in the occipito-posterior position, and the limbs will be felt more close to the midline on the left side of the abdomen.

Palpation: Leopold's manoeuvre (Figure 6.3) includes the various grips described below.

The initial assessment starts with the *fundal height* expressed in weeks of gestation. This is important to alert about growth-restricted fetuses as well as large babies.

Symphysio-fundal height: The uterine height in centimetres can be used for objective documentation and for calculating the fetal weight.

Palpating the part of the fetus in the fundus (*fundal grip*) of the uterus should be done with the palm and fingers to note down the lie and the possible presentation.

Lateral grips reveal the back of the fetus. Knowing the back of the fetus and hence the position of the occiput is important information for contemplating assisted vaginal delivery in case needed. Also, it helps to localize the fetal heart. The palm is moved from the fundus down to appreciate the uniform curved resistance suggestive of the back on one and the knobby irregularities on the

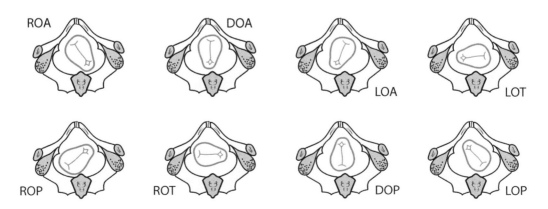

FIGURE 6.2   Various positions in vertex presentation.

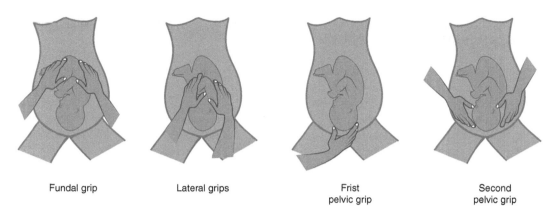

| Fundal grip | Lateral grips | Frist
pelvic grip | Second
pelvic grip |

FIGURE 6.3   Diagram depicting Leopold's manoeuvres.

opposite lateral grip suggestive of the limbs. Adequate liquor helps in the delineation of the limbs. The back position about the midline gives a clue to the position of the fetus. When the back is closer to the midline, the occiput is likely to be anterior. In the occipito-transverse position, the back is more towards the side of the abdomen, and in the occiput-posterior position, the back will be far out in the flanks. The fetal limbs are felt easily close to the midline on the left side in the right occipito-posterior position.

The *first pelvic grip* (*Pawlik's grip*) exam is done by placing the examiner's ulnar border of the right hand on the upper border of the pubic symphysis of the patient and holding the presenting part with the fingers and the thumb. A hard globular part suggests the head, and a firm part suggests breech. It is likely to be empty in the shoulder presentation. If the felt part is ballotable, it is unengaged.

For the *second pelvic grip*, the obstetrician should face the feet of the patient. The palms are placed on either flank and slowly moved down to the level of the inguinal ligament. Now raise the heels of the palm to allow the fingers to palpate deeper for the poles of the head.

The second pelvic grip is omitted in the breech presentation but gives valuable information in the cephalic presentation. The palpation of the two bony landmarks, occiput at the side of the back and the sinciput on the opposite side, confirms that it is vertex presentation. The sinciput feels more distinctly compared to the occiput. In a situation like a face or a brow presentation, the sinciput will not be palpable, and there will be a groove between the back and the occiput. In vertex presentation, the relation of the levels of occiput and sinciput to the pubic symphysis reflects on the level of deflexion. In the well-flexed head, the sinciput is at a higher level than the occiput. Diverging hands in the second pelvic grip suggest an engaged head. If the hands converge, then the head is not engaged. In the occipito-posterior position, the head is likely to be deflexed.

Thus, the following information can be obtained by the second pelvic grip:

- Confirm the presentation.
- Determine the presenting part.
- Determine the attitude of the head.
- Determine if the head is engaged or not.

In a labouring woman, the above findings should be carefully noted. The fifths of the head palpable above the pelvic brim during the first pelvis grip should also be noted down. This assessment is made by the number of fingers that can hold the head above the brim during the first pelvic grip.

If only the sinciput is palpable in the second pelvic grip, then the station can be expected to be around "−1" or "0".

We should also note down the uterine contractions for their frequency, intensity, duration, and the tone of the uterus between the contractions.

Last but not least is the *assessment of the baby's weight*. This can be done by various formulae like the *Johnsons, Dare, and Dawn's method*.

Johnson's formula: Fetal weight in grams [1] = 155 × (fundal height in cm − K), K = 11 (fetal head at plus stations), K = 12 (fetal head at zero station), and K = 13 (fetal head at minus stations). One has to subtract one from the fundal height for women weighing more than 90 kg.

Dare's formula [2]: Fetal weight in grams = fundal height in cm × abdominal girth in cm.

The Dare's method also takes into account the width of the subcutaneous tissue by callipers.

These are based on clinical measurements and may only give an approximation. Every obstetrician should learn to assess the clinical estimate based on the various grips and the overall volume occupied. Ultrasound assessment by Hadlock's formula gives the most accurate value. However, the same may not be possible in all pregnancies in busy labour rooms.

Auscultation: The fetal heart sounds are best heard across the back of the fetus as the flexed upper limbs occupy the front. Thus, the middle of the spino-umbilical line is the best location to listen to the fetal heart sounds in the occipito-anterior positions. The sounds should be noted for the rate as well as the rhythm or the regularity. The examiner's left hand should be on the maternal radial pulse to ensure that the sounds heard on the abdomen are different from the maternal pulse rate.

The fetal heart sounds are heard as distinct lub dub sounds. In occipito-transverse and occipito-posterior position, the sounds are the best-heard way out in the mother's flanks that have the fetal back. In occipito-posterior positions, sometimes the fetal heart sounds may be heard in the opposite side close to the midline across the chest of the fetus.

The additional sounds that can be heard on auscultation are called souffle. The uterine souffle is the pulsations across the uterine artery. These correspond to the maternal heart rate and are heard usually on the sides of the abdomen. The funic souffle is the sound transmitted from the umbilical cord through the amniotic fluid to be heard across the abdominal wall. These may vary in their position and correspond to the fetal heart rate. The souffle is heard as a "whoosh" sound. During labour, the location of the fetal heard sounds keeps changing and progressively moves lower down on the maternal abdomen with the descent of the fetus in the pelvis. The sounds also shift from the spino-umbilical line to the midline with rotation of the back during labour. Keenly observing these changing positions in the fetal heart location also gives an idea of the cardinal movements of the fetus during labour.

MECHANISM OF LABOUR

Fetal journey through the maternal pelvis to the outside world uses a lot of science, and the fetus has the inherent intelligence to steer itself through the pelvis.

The events during this journey involve many cardinal steps.

It is important to keep in mind a few facts.

- The commonest position is LOA (vertex presentation).
- The transverse and the oblique diameter are more than the anteroposterior diameter at the inlet of the maternal pelvis.
- The levator ani muscle attaches at the ischial spines' level and is directed downwards, forwards, and medially.
- The maximum diameter at the outlet of the pelvis is the anteroposterior diameter.

This means that the fetus must use the oblique or the transverse diameter at the inlet to negotiate its longitudinal head diameter (explained below) and must rotate to bring its longitudinal diameter to the AP diameter of the outlet. The direction of the levator ani muscles helps in rotating the pole that touches it first to a midline direction.

The longitudinal diameter is dynamic and decreases with increasing flexion. The transverse diameters of the head, on the other hand, are by and large fixed.

MECHANISM OF LABOUR IN LOA POSITION

With the onset of labour and increasing uterine contractions, *progressive flexion and descent of the head* occur (Figure 6.4). The head gets *engaged*. The suboccipito-bregmatic is the longitudinal, and biparietal is the transverse *engaging diameter* of the fetus. The *diameter of engagement* in the pelvis is the right oblique diameter of the inlet of the pelvis. With further descent, the leading occiput reaches the pelvis floor muscle. It undergoes *internal rotation* towards the midline by 1/8th of a circle (45°) head movement to bring the sagittal suture (suboccipito-bregmatic diameter) in the anteroposterior diameter of the outlet of the pelvis. Thus, the neck sustains a torsion by 1/8th of a circle.

With further progress of labour and descent, when the cervix dilates fully, crowning occurs, and the *head is born by extension*. The occiput, the vertex, the sinciput, the forehead, and the face are born in that order. Once the head is born, it rotates back by 1/8th of the circle to undo the torsion sustained by the neck. This is called *restitution*. At this time, the shoulder (BisAcromiun diameter) that had engaged in the left oblique diameter of the inlet of the pelvis reaches the pelvic floor. The anterior shoulder reaches the pelvic floor first and gets rotated towards the midline. This manifests as further *external rotation* of the head so that the fetus faces the mother's right thigh in LOA position.

The anterior, followed by the posterior shoulder, is delivered. The trunk is delivered by *lateral flexion* at the spine. The bitrochanteric diameter of the buttocks engages in the left oblique diameter of the inlet of the maternal pelvis. The traction on the baby while delivering the shoulders automatically turns the bitrochanteric diameter to the anteroposterior diameter of the pelvis outlet, and the buttocks get delivered. The delivery after the shoulder is so quick that one may not get time to observe these mechanisms at the hip joint.

Thus, these movements are governed by the science of the pelvis's diameter and the fetus's ability to steer through smoothly. The pelvic floor tissue recoil further helps the fetus in steering its way out to the world.

Spontaneous good uterine contractions, average size of the fetus, favourable (occipito-anterior) position with good flexion, and adequate gynaecoid pelvis are the key to the smooth labour journey.

Progressive flexion at the atlantooccipital joint occurs naturally. The fulcrum (atlantooccipital joint) is close to the short arm (head), given the spine as the rigid linear arm that must negotiate. So when the short arm (head) leads the journey, the short arm must flex or extend completely on this long arm (the fetal spine) to continue the journey through the curved cylinder (the pelvis). The atlantooccipital joint is placed more posteriorly on the head, so flexing the head will be more intelligent to reduce the total length of the spine. Flexing is also favoured as the cylinder is longer posteriorly and shorter anteriorly.

The anterior part of the pelvis is as short as the length of the pubis symphysis. Anything that comes below the pubis symphysis is automatically born. The occiput comes under the pubis symphysis first and gets born. As soon as the occiput is released, the head gets the freedom to extend at the atlantooccipital joint. The sinciput, vertex, forehead, face, and lastly, the chin sweep across the sacrum and are born as the head extends.

MECHANISM IN RIGHT OCCIPITO-POSTERIOR POSITION

In the occipito-posterior position, the back (and hence the occiput) is posterior, and the sinciput is anteriorly placed. The broader biparietal diameter is posterior, and the narrower bitemporal diameter is anterior. The fetus might assume this position to adapt for the narrower forepelvis at the inlet, as would be seen in anthropoid pelvis and pelvis with android tendency.

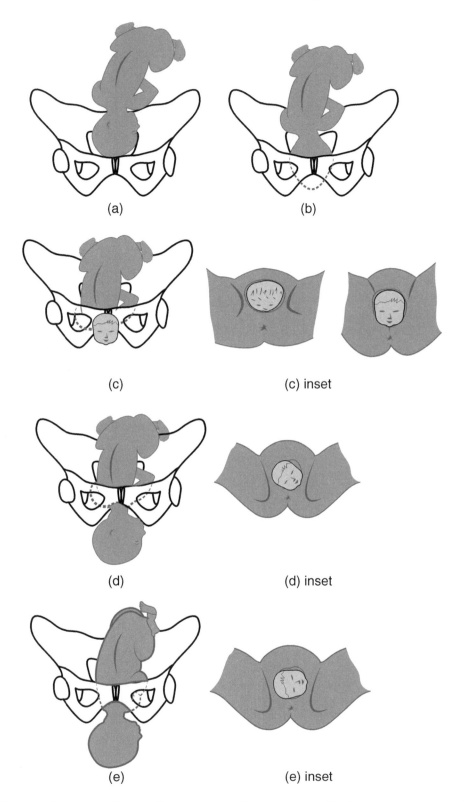

FIGURE 6.4 Mechanism of labour. The inset shows the movements of fetal diameters to maternal diameters: (a) ROA position; (b) internal rotation of head by 45°; (c) delivery by extension of the head; (d) restitution; and (e) external rotation.

The head is invariably deflexed, probably to adapt to the reverse curve of the maternal spine at the level of the upper back and neck of the fetus. So the occipito-frontal or the suboccipito-frontal diameter of the fetal head is the *engaging diameter. The diameter of engagement* in the maternal pelvis is the right oblique diameter of the inlet.

With progressive uterine contractions and continued flexion, the head reaches the pelvic floor. At the pelvic floor, any of the below four can happen:

a. *Complete anterior rotation* means that the occiput completely rotates to come under the pubis symphysis.
b. The occiput undergoes *short posterior rotation* to come to the sacrum in midline resulting in a direct occipito-posterior position.
c. There is no rotation, and it *persists as occipito-posterior.*
d. There can be incomplete rotation resulting in the right occipito-transverse position. If further progress gets arrested in the second stage, it is called *deep transverse arrest.*

Complete Anterior Rotation

This means the rotation is completed by 135° (3/8 circle) to bring the occiput under the pubic symphysis. The neck usually cannot sustain a 3/8 twist, so either

i. The neck twists by 1/8th of the circle and the 2/8 rotation is completed by shoulder rotation. The shoulders that had engaged in the left oblique diameter of the inlet of the pelvis rotate and come to occupy the right oblique diameter of the pelvic brim.
ii. The neck rotates by 2/8th and the shoulder by 1/8th of the circle.
iii. Rarely the neck itself undergoes a 3/8th rotation.

The first is the more common situation where the neck sustains only 45° torsion, and the bisacromial diameter that had engaged in the left oblique diameter of the inlet of the pelvis rotates to the right oblique diameter to complete the rest of the 2/8th rotation. The rotation occurs in the transition phase (from 8 cm onwards and during the second stage). Thus, the occiput comes under the pubic symphysis. With further descent and in the second stage, crowning occurs, and the head is born by extension. Once the head is born, there is restitution by 1/8th of the circle to undo the torsion in the neck. The bisacromial diameter which is now in the right oblique diameter rotates by 1/8th of the circle to occupy the anteroposterior diameter of the outlet. This is manifested as further external rotation of the head so that the newborn faces the left maternal thigh in the right occipito-posterior position. The anterior, followed by the posterior shoulder, is delivered.

The complete rotation usually is achieved in 90% of the cases. For complete rotation to occur, the following are necessary.

A. Good uterine contractions
B. A good amount of liquor in the hind waters for allowing shoulder rotation
C. Gynecoid pelvis
D. Average size fetus

Spontaneous Short Posterior Rotation by 45°

This results in a direct occipito-posterior position. This is more often seen in the anteroposteriorly oval (anthropoid) pelvis or pelvis with the high inclination – the bregma hinges behind the pubic symphysis. The longitudinal diameter of the head is likely to be suboccipito-frontal due to mild deflexion. The delivery in such a situation is called face to pubes delivery (also detailed in Chapter 13). The head is born by flexion to deliver the occiput and the vertex. Then the sinciput, the forehead, and the face of the fetus are delivered by extension. Restitution of the head occurs at 45° to undo the torsion on the neck. The anterior shoulder reaches the pelvic floor and undergoes rotation by 1/8th of a circle so that the bisacromial diameter occupies the anteroposterior diameter of the outlet of the pelvis. This is manifested as external rotation of the head to the left side so that in the right occipito-posterior position while undergoing face to pubes delivery, the fetus will look at the left thigh of the mother. The body is born by lateral flexion at the spine. The transverse biparietal diameter of the skull occupies the posterior part of the birth canal and distends the perineum. So the wider biparietal diameter, which is posterior towards the perineum, can cause tears involving the external anal sphincter and or the anal mucosa (complete perineal tears). A liberal 60° episiotomy and good perineal support are crucial to prevent complete perineal tears.

Persistent Occipito-Posterior Position

The head fails to rotate and persists in an occipito-posterior position. If the labour progresses and the head descends, then it can deliver as face to pubes spontaneously in women with the anthropoid pelvis. If there is a delay in the second stage and absence of features of cephalopelvic disproportion, then vacuum- or forceps-assisted delivery can be attempted to deliver the fetus as face to pubes. Caesarean section may be warranted in the pelvis with android tendency, features of disproportion causing non-descent, or in the presence of fetal heart rate abnormalities.

Incomplete Anterior Rotation of the Head by 1/8th of a Circle

In this situation, the suboccipito-frontal or occipito-frontal diameter occupies the transverse diameter of the obstetric outlet. This condition becomes "deep transverse arrest" when conditions are unfavourable and labour comes to a standstill. More about this is discussed in Chapter 13.

The time needed to complete the 270° rotation makes the labour prolonged in the occipito-posterior position and the ill fit of the deflexed head results in an elongated bag of the membrane that tends to rupture prematurely. Thus, it is important to keep the woman well hydrated and nourished. Changing her position to knee-chest or lateral position helps in rotation of the head and reduced perception of the back pain.

The cardinal movements of the head during labour can be appreciated by abdominal examination and digital vaginal examination. One needs to carefully note down the baseline admission findings to appreciate the changes as labour progresses.

REFERENCES

1. Johnson RW. Calculations in estimating fetal weight. *Am J Obstet Gynecol* 1957; 74: 929.
2. Dare FO, Ademoworw AS, Ifaturoti OO, Nganwuchu A. The value of symphysis fundal height/abdominal girth measurements in predicting fetal weight. *Int J Gynecol Obstet* 1990; 31: 243–248.

7 Management of Labour

Gowri Dorairajan
Jawaharlal Institute of Postgraduate Medical
Education and Research (JIPMER)

The onset of uterine contractions is the starting point for labour. They are perceived as pain by the woman. Labour pains can be true or false pains.

Prelabour, a few days to 1 or 2 weeks before labour, a woman may feel lightening. This is a feeling of lightness or relief in the upper abdomen as the head descends to fix or engage in the pelvis. This is more so in a primigravida. She may also experience backache frequently, along with slightly increased vaginal discharge. This is due to slightly enhanced Braxton Hicks contractions and the prelabour softening, effacement of the cervix (maturation of the cervix), and filling up of the lower segment by the presenting part.

FALSE LABOUR PAIN

These are ill-sustained uterine contractions perceived more often in the front of the lower abdomen. They are not regular and are inefficient in causing progressive cervical dilation and effacement. False labour pains may be exaggerated in a few, meriting admission a few days before the onset of true labour.

IDENTIFICATION OF TRUE LABOUR

Symptoms

True labour pains: The woman would experience pain that starts in the lower back, spreads to the front of the abdomen, and radiates to the thigh. This may be described as something like the cramps they used to feel during menstruation. True labour pains increase in duration, frequency, and intensity and occur at regular intervals starting once in half an hour and progressively become frequent enough to be once in 2 or 3 minutes. The woman may perceive it as a painful tightening. It is felt more as backache, to begin with, as the cervix is more resistant. But later, the abdominal component becomes more prominent. The posterior position of the fetus may tremendously increase the backache component. So persistent predominant backache in established labour forewarns about the posterior position of the fetus.

Show: Expulsion of mucus plug from the cervix along with blood staining is an important symptom accompanying labour pain and signifies opening up of the cervix. Sometimes it may be excessive, and women may emphasise this symptom as bleeding and less on the pain component. This exaggerated show may sometimes be confused as antepartum haemorrhage.

Signs of Labour

When a woman complains of pain and show, palpation of uterine contractions should confirm labour onset.

Uterine contractions: These are felt as hardening of the uterus on abdominal examination. One should make a note of the frequency, duration, and intensity of each contraction. Intensity is subjectively described as the ability to indent the uterus during a contraction. In moderate or good uterine contractions, the uterus cannot be indented. With experience, the perception of intensity becomes

DOI: 10.1201/9781003034360-7

easier by feeling the hardness of the uterus during a contraction without a need to indent it. The intensity should not be assessed based on the woman's groans and sighs of pain, as that varies based on the woman's pain threshold.

Progressive dilation and effacement of the cervix: The goal of labour is to deliver the fetus to the external world. This requires that the cervix dilates completely and the birth canal forms and the uterine contractions bring about progressive descent of the fetus. A progressive increase in effacement and dilation of the cervix noted on subsequent vaginal examination confirms that she is in labour.

Formation of the bag of membranes: This is felt like a bag filled with water (liquor) distal to the presenting part on internal digital examination. It characteristically becomes tense during uterine contractions and less pronounced when the uterus relaxes. This is a confirmatory sign of labour in the presence of uterine contractions.

ASSESSMENT OF A WOMAN IN LABOUR

Risk assessment: Whenever a woman is admitted to the labour ward, first it is important to review and document her history for the duration, intensity, frequency of pains, any passage of amniotic fluid/blood, perception of fetal movements, and any immediate problems such as bleeding, fever, and greenish discharge.

Second, we must establish the exact date to confirm the period of gestation. It is established with the last menstrual period date as well as the first scan.

The third step is to review her antenatal records for any risk condition, her blood investigation reports including blood group, any problems noted during the current pregnancy, and any coexisting medical morbidities.

EXAMINATION OF THE WOMAN

General physical examination: A thorough yet quick examination should be carried out to rule out risk problems such as anaemia, hypertension, obesity, and pyrexia. Systemic examination of the cardiovascular and other systems as guided by any specific complaints or any pre-existing disorders should also be carried out.

Baseline pulse should be noted.

Abdominal examination is carried out with the following goals:

A. **Rule out growth disorder**: Both growth restriction and macrosomia should be ruled out. The fundal height is noted. Any discrepancy with the period of amenorrhoea or the corrected period of gestation as calculated from the dating scan raises suspicion of a growth disorder.

B. **Know the presentation (detailed in Chapter 5)**: Leopold's manoeuvres should be done to know the presentation (first pelvic grip and fundal grip). The position of the back by is ascertained by the lateral grip. It is important to make a note of the back and position in early labour. In a cephalic presentation, the presenting part should be delineated in the second pelvic grip. Palpation of occiput on one side and sinciput on the opposite confirms that it is vertex presentation. The relation of the occiput and the sinciput to each other help in identifying flexion/deflexion of the head. The fifths above the brim should be noted (it reflects the extent of descent of the head into the pelvis).

One must remember that the first examination is the most valuable because as labour proceeds and liquor drains, it becomes difficult to establish the above information on abdominal examination. Late in labour contractions will obscure these findings and she may become less cooperative in the supine position, and if caput obscures the sutures on internal examination, it may become exceedingly difficult to know the position. Thus, I reemphasise that the first examination should specify these findings on abdominal examination.

C. **The weight of the baby**: Clinical estimation based on Leopold's grips is an easy and readily available method. One should make a note of the weight if a recent sonographic estimation is available. Estimation based on fundal height and abdominal girth measurements (Johnson's, Dare's, and Dawn's methods) may sometimes mislead and may under or over assess the weight. Sonographic estimation may not be practical for all patients admitted in busy labour rooms with high turnover. The estimation by clinical palpation is a skill that can be developed by estimating in all labouring women and corroborating it with the actual birth weight. The accuracy of estimation by clinical palpation can be improved with experience and feedback with actual birth weight.

D. **Liquor**: Clinical assessment of the amount of liquor should be noted. The assessment is based on the ease with which the parts of the fetus, especially the limbs, are palpated. Sometimes fetus can be seen to move the limbs (reflects adequate liquor). If facilities exist, then sonographic estimation should be done, and it is a good way to corroborate the clinical assessment with the sonographic assessment of the amniotic fluid index and improve the accuracy of clinical prediction.

E. **Fetal heart sounds**: It is important to note down the location of the heart sounds on abdominal examination. This gives a good confirmation of the likely position of the fetus. The location of the fetal heart sounds on the abdomen change from lateral to the midline and later down to the suprapubic region, with progressing labour. This reflects the dynamics of the cardinal movements of the fetus in labour. Besides location, it is also important to note down the rate and rhythm carefully. One must palpate maternal pulse with the non-dominant hand to confirm that the two are different and what is auscultated on the abdomen is indeed fetal sounds. This becomes a good checklist point when there is maternal tachycardia sometimes due to pyrexia. There have been instances where residents have confused the maternal souffle with the fetal heart because of the tachycardia and the rate sounding in the fetal heart range. Another important point is to continue to auscultate the fetal heart before and after a contraction to pick up any abnormal patterns related to the uterine contractions. Continued auscultation during contraction may be challenging as the woman moves around in pain and might prefer a different position Continued auscultations during contraction can reveal an abnormal pattern in relation to the timing of the contraction and help to harness the proficiency in detecting the type of decelerations even by auscultation. The technique for intermittent auscultation is detailed in Chapter 9.

Internal examination: This is a particularly important examination during labour. Strict aseptic precautions should be taken. The woman should be explained about the procedure to gain her cooperation, and all the findings should be noted down carefully and mindfully to avoid unnecessary repeat examinations. The internal examination helps us not only to confirm labour but also to know the stage of labour. It helps us pick up warning signals of abnormal labour. It is also an opportunity to confirm the position, observe the colour of the liquor, do the pelvic assessment, and it reveals a full rectum needing proper evacuation with an enema. The components to be noted down are listed below.

a. The cervical dilatation should be preferably expressed in centimetres and not fingers, even in early labour.

b. The cervical effacement is a rough approximation of the length of the cervix taken up and the length remaining expressed as centimetres or percentage.

c. The station of the head is the level of ischial spines is taken as zero station. The station is best expressed as −1 to −3 for the above ischial spine and +1 to +3 below the initial spine level. When expressed in centimetres, it is −1 to −5 and +1 to +5 cm, respectively above and below the level of ischial spines.

d. The status of the membranes is felt like a smooth lining over the head. The formation of a tense bag not only confirms labour but also confirms an intact membrane. In the absence of membranes, the roughness of hair will be felt when the fingers move in the opposite direction.

The position of the sutures. The sagittal suture will be palpated in vertex presentation running along in the middle of the field. When we follow the suture to its end, it will lead to the bregma or the lambda. Bregma is felt like a diamond-shaped membranous depression. The lambda is felt like a "y"-shaped bony depression. So, by locating the lambda and direction of the sagittal suture, it becomes easy to derive the position of the fetus. In a well-flexed vertex presentation, the bregma should not be palpated on vaginal examination.

e. One should note the colour of the liquor. Sometimes, when the head's station is low, one may have to slightly lift the head by sweeping the fingers beyond it to allow some hind water to escape. This may be necessary to ascertain the colour of liquor in certain situations.

f. Thereafter, a full pelvic assessment should be done to note down all points in detail (refer to Chapter 2)

We must document all the above findings at the admission of a woman in labour.

THE MANAGEMENT OF THE FIRST STAGE OF LABOUR

First stage of labour may last up to 11–12 hours. This could be a demanding time for the woman and the caregiver. Besides obstetric care, various aspects need attention.

a. **Admission**: Most women are advised to get admitted to the hospital once labour has been diagnosed. Depending on the proximity to the hospital, the health care system, and the hospital policy, some hospitals may admit low-risk women only in the active phase of labour.

b. **Part preparation and changing into hospital gowns**: This is driven by the hospital policy and the logistics of the setup. Part preparation by shaving or clipping helps in a better field of work while making and repairing episiotomy. Clipping of hair can also serve the same purpose. Changing into a hospital gown (the idea is to provide a clean gown and uniformity of dress in a common labour room of a public setup) again depends on the logistics and hospital facilities and the population's customs.

c. **Enema**: A low enema to activate the rectum is necessary if the rectum is full. It prevents soiling of the field at the time of delivery and helps in the good progress of labour. An empty rectum and urinary bladder become imperative at a second stage as she will tend to evacuate these organs on the table before the fetus can be pushed out.

d. **Ambulation and position**: A woman should be allowed to ambulate and assume the position of her choice and comfort during the first stage of labour. Women restricted to the bed find it more difficult to bear the pain. Squatting, knee-chest position, and the lateral position are more comfortable for the woman and also help in the progress of labour by improving the alignment of the head to the pelvic cavity.

e. **Diet and nutrition**: Labour is a very strenuous exercise. It is particularly important to provide adequate fluids and calories to the woman. Also, some tend to vomit when the cervix starts dilating, thereby further increasing the requirement. The concerns of a full stomach if anaesthesia is required for an emergency caesarean section may compel restricting the intake to a fluid diet. The woman should be encouraged to take plenty of fluids, juices, soup, a semi-solid diet like porridge, etc. In my observation, women who have been admitted right from latent phase or are being induced with poor Bishop score or have been in early labour for a long time do marvellously well when allowed to eat light meals, bath, and move around freely. It is important to prevent dehydration and exhaustion.

f. **Pain relief**: It is essential to provide some form of pain relief – the woman who has gone through birth preparedness classes, yoga, and breathing exercises in the prenatal period have better pain tolerance. Pharmacological and other non-pharmacological methods may be required to relieve pain. Yoga, breathing exercises, and music therapy have been shown to reduce pain. More of this is covered in Chapter 8.

g. **Birth companion**: With the LaQshya guidelines in place in India, a birth companion is being allowed even in the government setups with a heavy turnover of labouring women. Birth companion of women's choice should be encouraged. The birth companion needs to be oriented about the dos and don'ts and screened for common communicable diseases and their health before they are allowed.

h. **Emotional support**: Labour is a demanding period. The woman is not only in pain but also concerned about her fetal well-being. She may be extremely anxious, tense, and sometimes the pain makes them irritable and even violent. Antenatal birth preparedness classes help to allay anxiety in labour. Continued support from the birth companion as well as midwife and obstetrician is important. Frequent communication, reassurance about the progress of labour, and the fetal well-being goes a long way in gaining the cooperation and trust of women. She should feel secure and safe. There should be "respectful, dignified, consented, confidential, nondiscriminatory and nonjudgmental care imparted" (LaQshya guidelines).[1]

"A tense mind is a tense cervix". Allaying anxiety and fear ensure faster progress of labour. This will also discourage premature bearing down. A positive mindset for vaginal delivery, listening to music or watching television, etc. help in smoother and faster progress of labour. The obstetrician in charge should always make it a point to discuss the plan of labour, the progress of labour, and fetal condition with the woman and the relatives. This makes them feel better and under control. We should also involve them in decision-making. Good documentation of the counselling is also important.

i. **Antibiotics**: Routine administration of antibiotics to all is not necessary. An individualised decision must be taken for antibiotics. Hospital antibiotic policy should be followed.

MONITORING OF THE FIRST STAGE OF LABOUR

Monitoring: Diligent monitoring of the maternal and fetal condition and the progress of labour is the cardinal part of labour management. Partograph gives a quick overview of all these three aspects. Signs of abnormal labour are discussed in Chapter 10.

Monitoring during the first stage includes monitoring the well-being of the woman, the progress of labour, and the well-being of the fetus. Graphic representation of all three of the above in a single sheet – a "partogram" – has been used for many years. It makes the documentation and comprehension of the temporal change in findings during labour extremely easy to refer to at one glance. A partogram is a good objective tool to monitor a woman in labour.

The partogram:

a. This is a one-page graphic chart. The upper part of the chart contains patient identifying information. It also includes information on her parity and time of rupture of membranes (Figure 7.1a and b).

b. The upper part of the graph includes the plotting of the fetal heart rate on the Y-axis, with the X-axis representing time (each small box represents half an hour). The fetal heart rate is represented as a dark dot and joined to make a line. Below is the information on the colour of liquor represented as C/M/B for clear meconium and blood stained, respectively. If membranes are intact, "I" is written in the box. Next is information on moulding (further grading is detailed in Chapter 10).

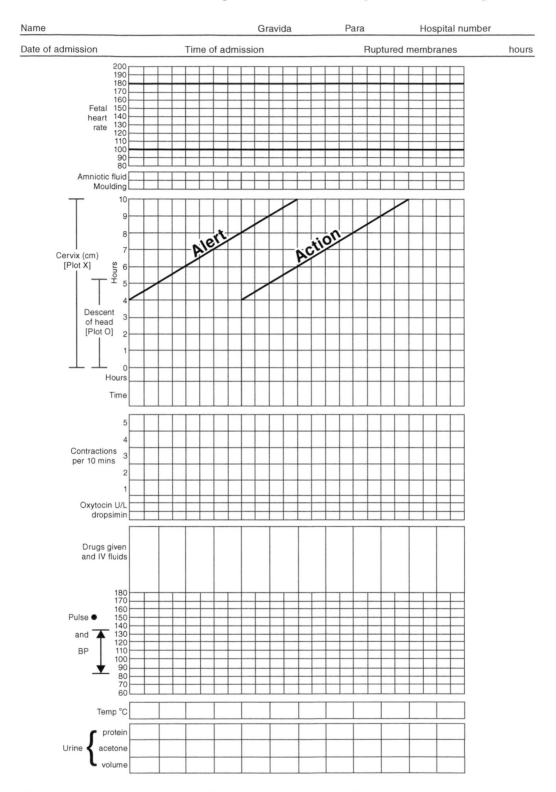

FIGURE 7.1A WHO partogram 2008. (Reproduced with permission from publication World Health Organization (2008) Managing Prolonged and Obstructed labour http://whqlibdoc.who.int/publications/2008/9789241546669_4_eng.pdf.)

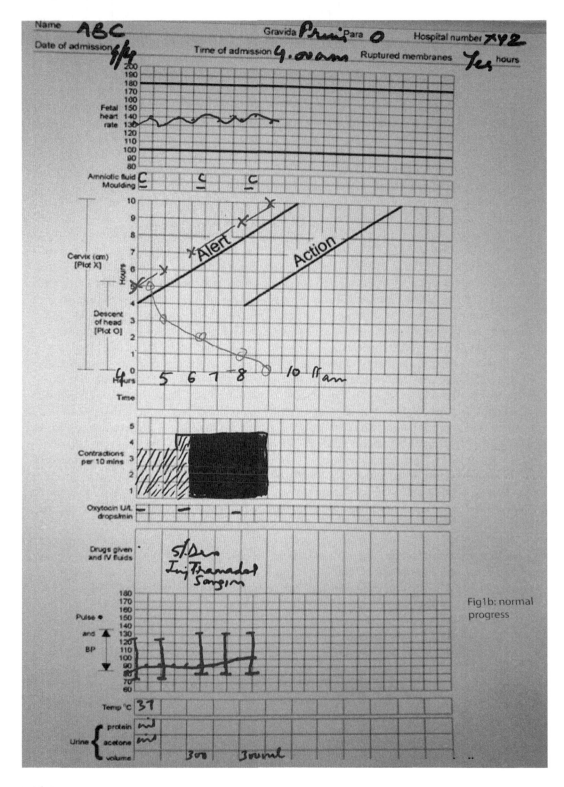

FIGURE 7.1B Case scenario partogram.

c. The next aspect is representing the progress of labour. This aspect of the partogram has undergone a lot of changes. The original partogram advocated by the WHO in 1994[2] included the latent phase of up to 8 hours and the active phase starting at 3 cm dilation also. However, WHO revised the partogram in 2008.[3] The latent phase was dropped, and the 4 cm dilation was considered the start of an active phase of labour. There are two lines already drawn and labelled as alert and action lines. The alert line is drawn starting from 4 cm dilatation. It is a line representing cervical dilation in centimetres and drawn at the rate of 1 cm/hour till 10 cm to obtain a straight line. The "X"-axis denotes time. Each box represents 1 hour, and the "Y"-axis represents 1 cm, each from 0 to 10 cm. So the alert line extends from 4 to 10 cm at the rate of 1 cm/. The action line is drawn 4 cm to the right of the alert line and parallel to it. The descent of the head is marked in the Y-axis, as shown in the partogram. It can alternatively be marked on the right side of the chart on the "Y"-axis from −5 to +5 cm (again 10 cm total).

Once the woman is in active labour, the dilation of the cervix at admission is marked on the alert line with an "X". The change of cervical dilatation against the time is also marked with an x. The x is joined to get the partograph of the labouring patient. The graph of cervical dilatation of the woman so obtained is read with the alert and action lines. The descent of the head is marked with an o corresponding with the admission station on the partogram sheet. The "o"s are joined to obtain the line that represents the descent of the head. The descent of the head will be a reverse curve proceeding from higher (minus) to lower (plus) stations (centimetres).

d. The next aspect of the partogram is the representation of uterine contractions. Both the intensity and the frequency can be recorded in the boxes provided. Mild contractions and those less than 20 seconds are represented as dotted points. Those between 20 and 40 seconds are represented as striated lines, and good contractions of more than 40 second duration are represented as a completely blackened-out box. There are five boxes placed vertically. The number of boxes shaded represents the number of contractions in a 10 minute window. The boxes shaded with dots/striated lines or completely darkened represent the intensity and duration of the contraction.

e. The next component of the partogram is designated for oxytocin infusion dose. The other drugs and intravenous fluids, including antibiotics and sedation, should be marked and the time they were administered is in the columns below the contractions.

f. The lower part of the partogram shows the maternal conditions like the **pulse** (marked as dark dots) and **blood pressure** plotted as vertical lines with the upper limit of the line at systolic and the lower limit of the line at diastolic blood pressure, as shown in the partograph. The maternal **temperature**, the **volume of voided urine**, and the presence of **proteins or ketones** in the urine should be marked in the lowermost part of the partogram. This completes the comprehensive graphic one-page representation of the progress of labour and fetal and maternal conditions.

The sample partogram of a primary gravida named ABC, who had rupture of membranes at 2:00 am and was admitted at 4:00 am on the 4 April 2019 in active labour, is shown in the figure. As is seen, the fetal heart remained normal, the liquor was clear, and there was no moulding. The progress of the labour graph remained to the left of the alert line. The head, which was at −3 station descended progressively, and she delivered uneventfully.

INTERPRETATION OF THE PROGRESS OF LABOUR GRAPH

The dilation graph of the labouring woman needs to be interpreted with the already marked alert and action lines. If the graph of labour of the woman is to the left of the alert line, it is a reassuring feature that labour is progressing normally. On the other hand, if the graph of the woman crosses to the right of the alert line, it suggests slow or abnormal progress of labour and cautions the care provider.

Caution alert line is crossed.

If the cervical dilatation graph of the patient proceeds to the right of the alert line, it is a warning signal. The graph of the progress of labour by cervical dilatation and descent of the head has to be interpreted along with other features such as moulding, the colour of the liquor, fetal heart rate pattern, and uterine contractions. As the name indicates, the alert line alerts the midwife and obstetrician. If the partograph of the woman crosses to the right of the alert line, then one must reassess carefully. One needs to relook at the fetus's estimated weight, position, and station. One should assess for the moulding and caput, colour of liquor, and fetal heart rate pattern. If the contractions are suboptimal and there is no evidence of pelvic disproportion, then augmentation with oxytocin may be necessary. The features suggestive of disproportion and dysfunctional uterine contractions are detailed in Chapters 10 and 11. Oxytocin, improving hydration with intravenous fluids, sedation, pain relief, and artificial rupture of membranes are a few of the measures that can be instituted. Even after taking these measures and observing for progress, if the labour graph does not proceed favourably and remains to the right and crosses the action line, it is a matter of great concern and needs termination by caesarean section or a second opinion from an experienced obstetrician. When the graph crosses the action line, there is protraction or arrest of labour. This is associated with a higher risk of operative delivery, fetal hypoxia and its sequel, and maternal problems like postpartum haemorrhage and sepsis.

CHANGING CONCEPTS IN THE DEFINITION OF ACTIVE LABOUR

The hallmark of active labour is that the cervical dilation proceeds at 1 cm/hour thereafter. The definition of the active phase of labour has undergone many changes since the introduction of the partograph in 1994. Initially, 3 cm dilation was taken as the beginning of active labour. But it was observed that labour doesn't accelerate by 1 cm/hour in many women even after achieving 3 cm dilation. Therefore, the definition changed to 4 cm in 2008. Zang observed labour progress and laid down his guidelines.[4] With rising caesarean section globally and nonprogress of labour being a frequently recognised indication for caesarean section, the Consortium of Labour[5,6] has redefined 6 cm as the start of the active phase of labour. Therefore, 6 cm dilatation is mandated to have been achieved before one can terminate by caesarean section for lack of progress. This initiative reduces the caesarean section rates for nonprogress of labour when the fetal condition is reassuring, and there are no features of cephalopelvic disproportion.

The partogram is an essential reference tool for all primary health care setups. It is also a decision tool for referral units. The limitations of the partogram are that the endpoint is taken as full dilation. Also, the interpretation of the assessment and the plan for further action is not documented in the partogram. Recently (2019), the WHO[7] has introduced a new generation partogram and labour care guide. The definition of the active phase of labour has been revised to 5 cm. This next-generation partogram also details the time and duration of the second stage of labour and the events therein. This partogram has seven sections. The first section identifies the patient and describes the labour characteristics. The second section details the supportive care provided to the woman in the form of birth companion, pain relief strategy, or any oral fluids or diet given to the woman. The third section is for recording the fetal heart pattern and other features like caput moulding and liquor colour. The fourth section provides details of the condition of the woman and information about her pulse, blood pressure, urine output, etc. The fifth section details the progress of labour. It mentions the number of hours spent at a particular dilation or station. The sixth section details the intravenous drugs, medication, and oxytocin administration. The seventh and the last section details the interpretation of assessment of the case and provides provision for detailing the plan of the index woman in labour. Recently e-partogram has been tested. It is an android tablet-based application. It provides auditory reminders and alerts about findings. It has been tested in Kenya, Tanzania, and Zanzibar.[89]

The interpretation of partograph should be made with caution in a grand multigravida or women with high risk like previous caesarean section and induced labour.

FREQUENCY OF MONITORING

It is essential to document all the findings in a woman in labour at admission as described in the partogram. The frequency of monitoring depends on the stage of labour.

The maternal condition: This needs to be monitored at least once in 4 hours in the latent phase and early labour if baseline findings were reassuring. The monitoring should include pulse, blood pressure, respiratory rate, temperature, hydration status, and the number of times and the volume of urine voided. The pulse rate may require hourly monitoring in the active phase of labour.

Progress of labour: Monitoring of the progress of labour can be done by abdominal examination and internal examination. The descent of the head is monitored as the fifth of the head above the brim or the number of poles palpable above the brim. The distance from the base of the skull to the highest point of the vertex in a well-flexed head is around 9 cm. Therefore, every fifth roughly represents 2 cm on this base-vertical distance. The location of the fetal heart shifts further down and towards the midline closer to the pubic symphysis. It is particularly necessary to monitor the contractions. The contractions should be observed for their frequency duration and intensity and expressed as duration/intensity/frequency or plotted in the partogram. This can be easily achieved by clinical palpation for most women. The caregiver should patiently spend time and wait for the contraction. The woman's expression of pain as groans or screams should not be taken as a criterion for monitoring contraction. Quite a few juniors tend to do that. The contractions need to be monitored every 2 hours in early labour and every hour in late labour. In women undergoing induction or augmentation, one should monitor the contractions every half an hour to help titrate the oxytocin drip to achieve the target contractions. An external tocodynometer can mislead depending on how tight or loose the contact of the probe is to the fundus of the uterus.

The vaginal examination should be documented in detail at admission. In low-risk women, repeat vaginal examination may not be needed more frequently than once in 4 hours. However, in some situations, it may have to be done within 2 hours to note down the progress, especially after the active phase of labour is reached. In early labour and latent labour, frequent vaginal examination should be avoided to prevent intrapartum infection. One must note all the findings, as mentioned earlier, during each vaginal examination. It is important to comment on caput, the position, and station in every subsequent digital vaginal review. These are dynamic findings like the dilatation of the cervix and subject to change as labour progress. Every vaginal examination should also comment on the colour of liquor and any abnormal findings such as asynclitism and coning (detailed in Section 7.2). Following pelvic assessment at the baseline examination, one should flag an alert if the pelvis appears borderline at any level and requires reexamination. A more thorough evaluation of the pelvis is again needed during the subsequent vaginal examination if the progress is abnormal after reaching the active phase (detailed in Section 7.2).

Fetal monitoring, the frequency, and the methods and details of monitoring is discussed in Chapter 9.

SECOND STAGE OF LABOUR

The second stage of labour is defined as the stage from full dilation of the cervix until the fetus's birth. It is a crucial period for the fetal journey.

IDENTIFICATION

The second stage has an active phase with the women getting the urge to push and a passive phase or descent phase where the cervix is fully dilated, but there is no urge to push. This will happen if the station is higher than the pelvic floor level. The passive phase can only be diagnosed by digital internal examination. The cervix is fully dilated and no longer felt on digital vaginal exam. The station of the head should be noted down. The expulsive phase or the pushing phase of the second stage is identified when a woman is seen bearing down, face flushed, expressing the pushing effort. The neck will show the veins appearing prominent. The perineum is seen bulging, the head is seen at the introitus, and the anal orifice appears open and stretched. Even in the second stage of labour, it is important to do an abdominal examination to ensure that no pole of the fetus is palpable because sometimes what is seen at the outlet or felt on digital review may be only a large caput. So, one must note down for caput formation and assess the lower strait of the pelvis for adequacy. This will help us ascertain to a fair degree as to which woman is likely to deliver without much assistance and which woman would require an operative vaginal delivery.

Maternal and fetal monitoring: The second stage is very crucial for maternal and fetal outcomes. The fetal heart needs to be monitored every 5 minutes. The maternal pulse may have to be monitored every half an hour or 15 minutes depending on the baseline pulse, underlying medical condition, induction or augmentation of labour, and any other risk condition.

Conduct of delivery: Once the second stage is confirmed and delivery is imminent in the active phase, the woman is brought to the edge of the table. At the time of delivery of the fetus, the position assumed by the mother can be dorsolithotomy, lateral, or squatting, depending on the woman's preference. The obstetricians prefer the lithotomy or dorsolithotomy position of the woman as most of the training is imparted in this position, and it is easy to observe the events and assist in this position.

It is essential to teach a woman how to bear down actively and breathe during the second stage. If intervention in the form of operative-assisted vaginal delivery is contemplated, consent (verbal) must be obtained after counselling and discussion about benefits and likely risks.

The five "C"[10]: Clean room, clean surface and table, clean hands, clean cord cut, and clean cord ties are important steps to be followed to reduce sepsis. The vulva and perineum and the abdomen below the umbilicus are cleaned with an antiseptic solution. This is critical to reducing infection.

The vagina is cleaned with an antiseptic solution. There is no need to catheterise women during the second stage routinely. She can still be encouraged to void in a bedpan.

Two recent meta-analysis[11,12] have suggested that warm compresses and massage of the perineum might reduce third- and fourth-degree tears. Also, the hands-off technique had fewer episiotomies, but data on other perineal trauma were insufficient.

A hands-on technique includes flexing the head, supporting the perineum, and aiding in slow slipping out of the head. Later, lateral flexion to deliver the shoulder is carried out to protect the perineum.

Performing an episiotomy at the peak of a contraction at crowning is decided when the perineum stretch threatens to tear the fourchette. The use of episiotomy should be **restrictive**.[13] If indicated, episiotomy is made when crowning has occurred. Crowning refers to seeing the head at the introitus without retracting the labia, even in the relaxed uterine phase. The angle of episiotomy at crowning should be 60° from the midline, and mediolateral is the preferred episiotomy.

Modified Ritgen manoeuvre: Once the occiput is born by flexion of the head, the obstetrician's hand should exert forward pressure on the chin through the perineum in front of the coccyx. The other hand, should exert pressure superiorly on the occiput (Figure 7.2). Next, the perineum is slowly slipped off the chin to ensure slow delivery of the head by extension. This helps in manual protection of the perineum and is likely to do away with the need for an episiotomy. The occiput is born under the pubic symphysis by flexion. This is followed by the birth of the vertex, the sinciput, the forehead, and the face by extension.

Once the head is born, one should allow spontaneous restitution to occur. Wipe and clean the face as one waits for external rotation of the head. So, the face which was looking at the perineum now faces the opposite thigh. The hands support the temporal aspect. The fingers are resting on the chin and occiput on either side of the neck. Gentle downward traction (lateral flexion) will deliver the

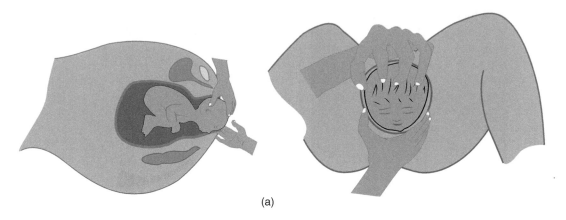

(a)

FIGURE 7.2A   Ritgen manoeuvre and manual protection of perineum in lateral and caudal view.

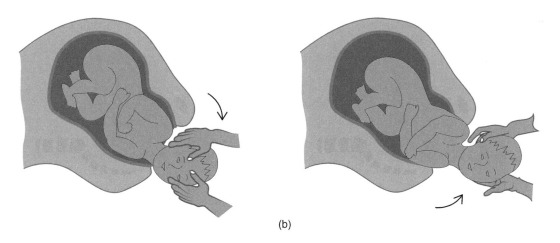

(b)

FIGURE 7.2B   Delivery of the shoulders.

anterior shoulder. Then the posterior shoulder is delivered by lifting the head upwards (Figure 7.2b). The trunk thus gets delivered by lateral flexion at the spine. The hands of the obstetrician should be repositioned with the right hand firmly holding the chest from under the posterior axilla and the other supporting the trunk and the anterior hip with the fingers up to the thigh. This ensures a firm hold on the newborn that may be slippery due to the vernix and the liquor. The newborn should never be held upside down. The new guidelines[14] discourage milking the blood from the cord to the fetus. They do not advocate holding the baby below the level of the placenta.

The face of the newborn is cleaned. The oropharynx is cleared of any secretions. There is no need for routine suctioning of the nasopharynx. Delayed cord clamping (after 3 minutes) is recommended. The cord is cut between the clamps after the pulsations stop unless there is a need for early clamping. The newborn can be landed on the mother's abdomen, and immediate rooming-in should be encouraged and recommended. This not only improves bonding but also reduces hypothermia and encourages early feeding. The oxytocin released on sucking further ensures good uterine contractility. However, logistics are to be kept in mind. The mother should be fully awake and in control and an assistant should ensure the baby does not fall off the mother's abdomen or chest.

MANAGEMENT OF THE THIRD STAGE OF LABOUR

The signs of placental separation have been detailed in Chapter 4. One must wait for the signs of placental separation before delivering the placenta. The uterus runs a risk of getting inverted if the cord is pulled with the placenta still attached to it. So the traction on the cord to deliver the placenta should be attempted only after one is sure that the placenta has got separated.

Conduct of placental delivery: The physiological management where the placenta is expelled automatically without any assistance by cord traction or uterotonics is no longer preferred. Active management is preferred. Once the signs of placental separation have been confirmed, the placenta is ready to be delivered. The method used is **controlled cord traction** (Figure 7.3). The umbilical cord is held in the right (dominant) hand (if long, it can be twined around the palm to give comfortable working length from the vagina and give firm steadiness while pulling). Steady traction is made first downwards, then parallel to the ground, and then forwards in the last part (in line with the curve of Carus). The cord traction should be applied only with counter traction by the opposite hand. The opposite is placed at the suprapubic part of the abdomen above the placental bulge. This hand should push the upper segment upwards and backward (counter traction) as the placenta is being pulled down (traction). The membranes follow the placenta. To prevent tearing of the membranes and to ensure their complete removal, one can slowly rotate the delivered placenta around the trailing membranes or grasp the membranes with a ring or artery forceps and deliver them completely. The membranes completely cover the cotyledons as they are delivered. After delivery, one must examine the placenta. The membranes are everted to their anatomical position, and the cotyledon surface is exposed. Check that all the cotyledons are intact and the membranes are completely removed. The uterus should not be explored routinely for looking for retained cotyledons or membrane bits.

Fundal pressure (Crede's method) to deliver the placenta should be highly discouraged.

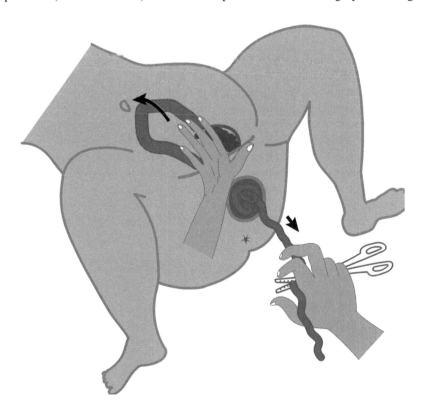

FIGURE 7.3 Line diagram showing controlled cord traction method of delivering the placenta.

Active Management of the Third Stage of Labour (AMTSL)

AMTSL is recommended by most societies, including the WHO, for every woman who is delivering to prevent postpartum haemorrhage. It can avoid atonic postpartum haemorrhage by 60%.

The **components of AMTSL** include administering a uterotonic agent at or after delivery of the fetus (avoid after the birth of the first child in multiple pregnancies), late cord clamping, and placental delivery by controlled cord traction. In addition, assessment of the fundus for tone is necessary, but routine fundal massage is not recommended any more.

Uterotonic agents used for AMTSL

Oxytocin: Ten units of oxytocin should be administered by intramuscular route, as soon as or within 1 minute of birth of the fetus. If the woman already has intravenous access, then the oxytocin can be given as an infusion (ten units in a bottle of ringer lactate) at 1–2 mL/minute. Intravenous bolus should be avoided as it can cause hypotension. The intravenous bolus dose should preferably not exceed five units and should be administered slowly over 1–2 minutes. Intravenous bolus is more often used in the controlled settings of caesarean delivery. In low resource countries, deliveries are conducted in the primary health centre or subcentre. Suppose there is a lack of trained personnel to administer drugs by parenteral route, **then uniject** (a preloaded sterile plastic softule containing ten unit oxytocin in a 1 mL solution with a sterile needle covered by a twist and break plastic cover) can be used. The advantage is that it can be administered even by untrained personnel with ease.

Misoprostol: This is recommended as an alternative. The advantage is that it is easily accessible, affordable, and can be administered by any route like oral/sublingual/rectal route, even by the community health workers or paramedical workers. Misoprostol can be stored at room temperature. Misoprostol of 600–800 µg has been advocated to be administered after childbirth. Misoprostol can cause fever and chills.

Carbetocin: An oxytocin analogue can be used as an alternative uterotonic. A dose of 100 micrograms is administered intramuscularly, slowly over a minute. Unfortunately, it is expensive and not readily available in all the countries. It has the advantage of not requiring a cold chain and a longer duration of action.

Ergometrine: Intravenous ergometrine 0.25 mg should be timed along with the delivery of the anterior shoulder and followed by slow delivery of the fetus. If the timing is not exact and gets delayed, it can cause retention of the placenta due to hourglass constriction of the uterus. In addition, it has more side effects like the sudden rise of blood pressure and spasms of arterioles. It should be avoided in hypertension, a woman with a history of migraine, and Raynaud's phenomenon. The advantage is a sustained tonic contraction of the uterus. It can also be given by intramuscular route. A combination of ergometrine 0.25 mg and oxytocin 5 units is used as an alternative in some countries.

Prostaglandin F2 alpha: 150 µg administered intramuscularly is not a preferred alternative. It can cause diarrhoea and is no longer used for the prevention of postpartum haemorrhage.

Administration of any one of the uterotonic is recommended for every childbirth to prevent postpartum haemorrhage. After completion of delivery, the fundus should be palpated for assessing the tone.

EPISIOTOMY

Refers to an incision made on the perineum, including the vagina, to enlarge the available space. It facilitates the delivery of the fetus.

The tissues cut are the vaginal wall, muscles of the perineum, and the overlying skin of the perineum.

Classification of episiotomies (Figure 7.4b): Though there are seven different types of episiotomy described[15] only four of them (enumerated below) are commonly practised in obstetrics.

Midline or median: This is a midline incision. The incision starts at midline or +3 mm of the midline. It is between 0° and 25° of the midline. This runs the risk of extension to involve the anal sphincter and the anal mucosa. When the need arises to deliberately extend it (for example, for unforeseen shoulder dystocia), there is a serious threat of injury to the anal sphincter and mucosa. Therefore, midline episiotomy is to be discouraged. Extension of the lower end transversely on the perineum can gain 2–5 cm and is called a modified median episiotomy.

Lateral: Incision starts laterally at least 10 mm away (or up to 2 cm away) from the midline and is directed towards the ischial tuberosity. It is limited by the groin fold and results in achieving only minimal extra space and cannot be extended if the need arises. This is also not practised. When a similar incision goes all the way around the rectum, it is called Schuchardt incision and is more often used in gynaecologic surgeries.

J-Shaped: This starts vertically down in the midline or within 3 mm for about 1–2 cm. After that, it is angled towards ischial tuberosity away from the anus in the midline. This is also not practised widely.

Mediolateral: Starting from the midline or within 3 mm and is directed well away from the midline at 60° towards the ischial tuberosity.

The ideal angle for mediolateral episiotomy is 60° from the midline. This ensures minimal risk of complete perineal tear. This angle can be ensured by using episcissors 60 or using an episometer.

The advantage of this episiotomy is the minimal risk of sphincter injury and the opportunity to deepen it or extend it safely when the need arises. The threat is that levator ani muscle may get involved when very deep. Vertical extensions may involve the lateral fornix and threaten the safety of the ureter during the repair. Also, the occurrence of supra levator hematoma in cases of extension of episiotomies is difficult to manage in the labour ward.

Anterior episiotomy is used in women with scarring due to genital mutilation in childhood.

The side of episiotomy: Most obstetricians are trained to stand on the foot end of the table. Right-sided episiotomies would appear convenient to make.

Most of the nurses and midwives are trained to stand by the woman's right side while delivering and find it convenient to make left mediolateral episiotomies. The side does not matter and is a matter of training and convenience and choice of the delivery personnel.

The author has a personal preference for right mediolateral episiotomy.

The episiotomy scissors: There are many episiotomy scissors such as Schumacher, Lawson Tait, and Waldmann. The Braun Stadler (Figure 7.4a) is the commonly used one. These are available in different sizes.

The scissors have angled or curved wide blades with a long shank. The shanks are flat to facilitate holding it at the ringed ends of the handle. It has a blunt, broad blade (sometimes knobbed at the tip). We can minimise the accidental injury to the anal or rectal mucosa beneath the vagina by the sharp end of the inner blade by keeping the shorter inner blade outer to the skin of the perineum (Figure 7.4c). The edges are bevelled to cut efficiently. One blade is longer than the other. The blades are set at an angle to the jointed shank.

Repair of the episiotomy (Figure 7.4d and e): The repair is done after completing placental delivery and exploring the genital tract to rule out any trauma or extension and higher degrees of perineal tear by rectal examination. Episiotomy is repaired in three layers. The repair starts with the vaginal mucosa. The first suture should be taken well above the visible apex (1 cm above) to prevent apex hematomas. The vessels are running vertically down, and the vessel's cut edge tends to retract beyond the apex. The vaginal mucosa is stitched continuously or locking in case of edge bleeding. The incised vaginal wall is sutured from the apex down to the mucocutaneous junction. The suture preferred is absorbable sutures like chromic catgut 0. The second layer approximates the perineal muscles (superficial and deep, transverse perineal muscles, and the bulbospongiosus muscle). This layer is sutured from side to side by interrupted sutures with chromic catgut ensuring approximation, obliteration of any dead space, and haemostasis. The skin can be sutured with subcuticular continuous sutures to reduce the number of knots protruding. Alternately, it can be approximated with vertical or horizontal mattress suture (with absorbable sutures like chromic catgut) with knots towards the lateral aspect to avoid faecal contamination. Though the angle of incision at the time of

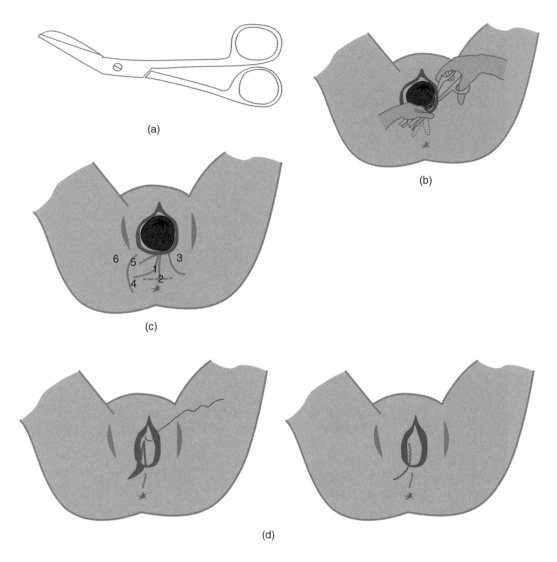

FIGURE 7.4   (a) Braun Stadler episiotomy scissors. (b) Line diagram showing the making of episiotomy. (c) Types of episiotomies: 1, median; 2, modified median; 3, lateral; 4, J-shaped; 5, mediolateral; and 6, Schuchardt incision. (d) Suturing the mucosa. (e) Repaired episiotomy wound (Redrawn from Kalis V, Laine K, de Leeuw J, Ismail K, Tincello D. Classification of episiotomy: towards standardisation of terminology. *BJOG* 2012;119:522–526.).

crowning is at 60°, but after suturing, the angle diminishes and the suture angle comes closer to the midline. If the knots are medial, they may become close to the midline and may tend to lodge the bacteria from faecal contamination if scrupulous hygiene is not maintained.

Role of rectal examination: The digital rectal examination should be done in all cases after vaginal delivery to rule out any sphincter tear even though the perineal skin may appear intact. It confirms the tear and helps in delineating the extent of anorectal mucosal involvement and ruling out buttonhole tears with an intact perineum. Keeping the index finger in the rectum and the thumb outside, a pill-rolling movement helps in delineating the disruption of the external and/or internal sphincter. The sphincter deficiency is recognised by the lack of tone of the external sphincter and the lack of rolling of tissue between the vagina and the rectal mucosa, indicating an internal sphincter injury. A missed internal sphincter injury would be the cause for flatus incontinence later.

A digital rectal injury after suturing of episiotomy may be necessary in some cases of upper or deep extension to exclude the inclusion of rectal mucosa in the suture bites.

Word of caution: While repairing episiotomies that have got extended upwards or into deeper planes or extended to include levator muscles, it is important to occlude all dead space.

The trick in such situations is to secure the apex of the vaginal mucosa first with a suture, thereafter with another suture, torn levator ani muscle on that side should be repaired. The dead space created lateral to the vagina should be approximated from the apex downwards before continuing with the vaginal mucosa. Suppose we attempt the deeper lateral layer after completing the mucosa. In that case, it becomes challenging to obliterate the depth of the deep lateral tunnel formed by the side along the length of the sutured vagina and the upper fibres of levator ani escape repair. This can result in haematoma formation high up in the dead space and also weakening of unrepaired levator muscle and predisposes to pelvic organ prolapse in the future.

A thorough cleansing of the vagina and the sutured skin site with an antiseptic solution like povidone-iodine is an excellent practice to minimise infection further.

A word of caution: Sometimes, a tampon is kept in the vagina to push the frilled cervix and reduce blood soiling the field for better visualisation and suturing of the apex. It is important to tag the tampon with gauze tape coming well outside the vagina. This will be a reminder to remove the tampon after the suturing is over. There are many instances of forgotten tampons as a cause for puerperal sepsis, especially in high turnover institutions. The author condemns the use of small gauzes for this purpose as they tend to slip into the posterior fornix. This may never show up on subsequent speculum examination as they are hidden in the posterior fornix, and the examiner gets falsely assured about the absence of gauze or tampon because the cervix is well visualised. Even on vaginal examination, it may escape attention because the fingers may not be inserted deep enough to reach the posterior fornix due to the discomfort of the episiotomy wound.

Routine use of antibiotics after a normal delivery is not necessary and can be judged as per the individual case or the hospital policy.

REFERENCES

1. *LaQshya*- Labour room quality improvement initiative, 2014 http://nhsrcindia.org/sites/default/-files/LaQshya-%20Labour%20Room%20Quality%20Improvement%20Initiative%20Guideline.pdf. Accessed on 15th March 2020.
2. WHO. Preventing prolonged labour: A practical guide. Geneva: WHO Division of Family Health, Maternal Health, and Safe Motherhood Programme. World Health Organization Maternal Health and Safe Motherhood Programme World Health Organization partograph in management of labour. *Lancet*. 1994c; 343:1399–1404
3. WHO. Managing prolonged and obstructed labour: Education materials for teachers of midwifery. In *Maternal Health and Safe Motherhood Programme. Education Material for Teachers of Midwifery: Midwifery Education Modules*, 2nd ed. World Health Organization. 2008. https://apps.who. int/iris/handle/10665/44145.
4. Zhang J, Troendle J, Mikolajczyk R, Sundaram R, Beaver J, Fraser W. The natural history of the normal first stage of labor. *Obstet Gynecol*. 2010; 115:705–710.
5. Bernitz S, Dalbye R, Zhang J, et al. The frequency of intrapartum caesarean section use with the WHO partograph versus Zhang's guideline in the Labour Progression Study (LaPS): A multicentre, cluster-randomised controlled trial. *Lancet*. 2019;393(10169):340–348. doi:10.1016/S0140-6736(18)31991-3.
6. Safe Prevention of Primary Caesarean Delivery. Obstetric Care Consensus. November1, 2014. ACOG Clinical Guideline.
7. WHO. *WHO Labour Care Guide: User's Manual*. World Health Organization; 2020. Licence: CC BY-NC-SA 3.0 IGO. Downloaded on 14th December 2020.
8. Litwin LE, Maly C, Khamis AR, et al. Use of an electronic partograph: Feasibility and acceptability study in Zanzibar, Tanzania. *BMC Pregnancy Childbirth*. 2018;18(1):147. doi: 10.1186/s12884-018-1760-y.

9. Sanghvi H, Mohan D, Litwin L, Bazant E, Gomez P, MacDowell T, Onsase L, Wabwile V, Waka C, Qureshi Z, Omanga E, Gichangi A, Muia R. Effectiveness of an electronic partogram: A mixed-method, quasi-experimental study among skilled birth attendants in Kenya. *Glob Health Sci Pract.* 2019;7 (4):521–539. doi: 10.9745/GHSP-D-19-00195. PMID: 31874937; PMCID: PMC6927834.

10. BirthModule. *5C Effective Perinatal Care (EPC) training package*, 2nd Edition. WHO Regional Office for Europe. 2015.

11. Aasheim V, Nilsen A, Reinar L, Lukasse M. Perineal techniques during the second stage of labour for reducing perineal trauma. *Cochrane Database Syst Rev* 2017; 6. Art. No.: CD006672. doi: 10.1002/-14651858.CD006672.pub3.

12. Aquino CI, Guida M, Saccone G, Cruz Y, Vitagliano A, Zullo F, Berghella V. Perineal massage during labor: A systematic review and meta-analysis of randomised controlled trials. *J Matern Fetal Neonatal Med.* 2020;33(6):1051–1063. doi: 10.1080/14767058.2018.1512574. Epub 2018 19th September. PMID: 30107756.

13. Jiang H, Qian X, Carroli G, Garner P. Selective versus routine use of episiotomy for vaginal birth. *Cochrane Database Syst Rev* 2017; 2:CD000081.

14. Aziz K, Lee HC, Escobedo MB, Hoover AV, Kamath-Rayne BD, Kapadia VS, Magid DJ, Niermeyer S, Schmölzer GM, Szyld E, Weiner GM, Wyckoff MH, Yamada NK, Zaichkin J. Neonatal resuscitation: 2020 American heart association guidelines for cardiopulmonary resuscitation and emergency cardio-vascular care. *Circulation.* 2020; 142(16_suppl_2):S524–S550 (ISSN: 1524–4539).

15. Kalis V, Laine K, de Leeuw J, Ismail K, Tincello D. Classification of episiotomy: Towards a standardisation of terminology. *BJOG.* 2012; 119:522–526.

8 Obstetric Analgesia

Chitra Chatterji and Atish Pal
Indraprastha Apollo Hospital

INTRODUCTION

Since ancient ages, childbirth has been recognised as one of the most painful human experiences. A wide array of management has been used over the years based on various cultural and religious beliefs and medical practices prevalent at that time. Early methods included therapies such as talisman, magic belts, and readings from the holy books, and later methods included pharmacological treatments like the use of sponges dipped in plant juices with sedative properties. Healthcare workers wishing to provide labour analgesia had to face a lot of social prejudices though severe, labour pain was considered physiological, self-limiting, and not detrimental to mother and newborn. Since most of the treatments carried significant risk to the mother and baby, thus a non-interfering approach was favoured.

In the past century, obstetric analgesia options have become much more effective and safer. However, false beliefs and controversies have always been associated with labour pain relief. Thus, provision of safe and effective pain-free labour has been a continuous struggle for everyone concerned. Nowadays, various trials, studies, and reviews have confirmed neuraxial analgesia as the technique of choice for labour analgesia.

HISTORY

In the 19th and early part of the 20th century, most pregnant women had to rely on neighbours and other local assistance for childbirth, and these attendants supervised labour and child delivery. For many years, various substances such as opioids, sedative potions, alcohol, and medicinal plants were used to relieve labour pain. James Young Simpson, in 1847, first used ether for stillborn delivery. Simpson also experimented with other potential anaesthesia agents and adapted the use of chloroform in labour as an anaesthetic agent.

Anaesthesia for childbirth was still not widely accepted. There was much discussion in the medical parleys about labour analgesia, mainly about the importance of pain in labour and the effects of various maternal and child health treatments. Simpson, Channing, etc. advocated that pain was not mandatory for the process of childbearing; therefore, it should always be relieved when possible. However, many others firmly believed that labour pain and childbirth were inseparable and suppressing labour pain in any way would inhibit the labour process.

This discussion wavered on till the late 19th century. Finally, however, educated women from well to do families had started expressing their desire for proper medical pain relief by qualified physicians. Queen Victoria was one such famous name who helped advocate labour analgesia by asking for pain relief during childbirth. She was administered chloroform through a handkerchief by Dr John Snow in 1853.

DOI: 10.1201/9781003034360-8

LABOUR PAIN AND PAIN PATHWAY

Mechanisms and Pathway

Labour is the period from the onset of painful uterine contractions till childbirth. Labour pain has two components: visceral and somatic (Figure 8.1).

Visceral Pain

The visceral component of labour pain is felt during the initial first and second stages of labour. Pressure gets transmitted to the cervix by contractions of the uterus and causes cervical stretching. This stretching of the cervical wall activates the nociceptive afferents, and these innervate the endocervical part and segments from T10 to L1.

Visceral pain is dull in nature and is usually localised to the lower abdominal, sacral, and back areas (T10–T12 dermatomes). Visceral pain usually shows a response to opioid analgesics.

Somatic Pain

In the late first and second stages of labour, fetal descent occurs through the birth canal. Descent causes stretching and damage to the pelvic, vaginal, and perineal tissues and manifests as the somatic component of pain and is transmitted by the A-delta fibres. As the descent progresses and cervical dilatation increases, the severity of pain also increases. The main nerves associated with the somatic pain of labour are pudendal nerve, perineal branch of posterior cutaneous nerve of thigh, branches of ilioinguinal, and genitofemoral nerves.

Somatic pain occurs close to delivery and is sharp and usually more resistant to opioid medications.

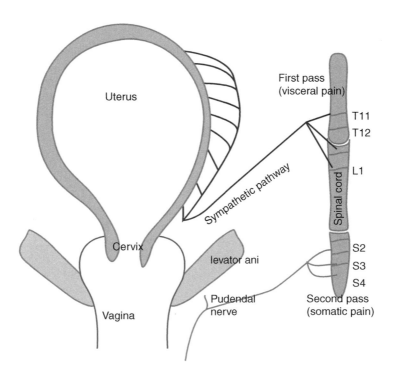

FIGURE 8.1 Line drawing showing the pain pathway.

TECHNIQUES OF LABOUR ANALGESIA

NON-PHARMACOLOGICAL METHODS

- Psychological methods
- Physical methods: hydrotherapy, effleurage, movement, and position changes
- Transcutaneous electrical nerve stimulation (TENS)
- Alternative methods: acupressure and hypnobirthing

PHARMACOLOGICAL METHODS

- Systemic analgesia: intravenous agents and inhalational agents
- Regional neuraxial techniques
- General anaesthesia

NON-PHARMACOLOGICAL METHODS

1. **Transcutaneous electrical nerve stimulation (TENS)**
   - Based on the "gate theory" of pain
     - Use of electrical stimulation
     - Two electrodes are stuck on the skin and connected to a battery-powered machine
     - The machine delivers small electrical current pulses to the body
     - Gives some amount of pain control
     - Can be used with other therapies
     - No harm to mother or baby
2. **Lamaze Breathing technique**
   - French obstetrician Fernand Lamaze pioneered Lamaze breathing
   - In the 1950s, he championed psychoprophylaxis to prepare pregnant women with physical and psychological training
   - This includes conscious relaxation and controlled breathing as an alternative to drugs to manage contraction pain during childbirth
   - Lamaze breathing is a breathing technique based on the idea that controlled breathing can decrease the perception of pain and enhance relaxation
3. **Immersion in water**
   - Sensation of warm water supports the gravid uterus and inhibits pain transmission
4. **Acupuncture**
   - Fixed points on the body are stimulated with very fine needles
   - May inhibit the transmission of pain or help in the production of natural endorphin
   - It is an invasive procedure and needs a trained individual
5. **Massage**
   - Mechanism is by inhibition of pain transmission
   - Also provides support and helps in distraction
6. **Waterblocks**
   - 0.1 mL of sterile water is injected over the sacral region in four spots
   - Procedure is easy to perform
   - Provides brief relief only (45–90 minutes)
7. **Hypnosis**
   - Entering a state of altered consciousness to change the pain perception
   - Appears to reduce the overall analgesic usage

PHARMACOLOGICAL METHODS

Inhalational Methods

1. **Entonox**: Consists of oxygen and nitrous oxide in a 50:50 mixture. As nitrous oxide has a low blood-gas solubility coefficient (0.47), the equilibration with blood is very fast and thus has a rapid wash off from the lungs. The patient should be trained regarding the proper and effective usage method. Fifty seconds or ten normal breaths are needed for optimal effect. Entonox can cause nausea, sedation, and even loss of consciousness in some patients. There is an increased risk of diffusion hypoxia and desaturation when Entonox is used in combination with meperidine.

   Entonox is usually administered through a cylinder (Figure 8.2a) in most institutes or via a piped apparatus. It is designed to be self-administered by the patient under medical supervision. When a patient inhales more than the required gas, she will become drowsy and subsequently drop the mask. The Entonox effect will wear off fast as the patient starts breathing room air. The attendant or healthcare provider should not hold the mask for the patient during use, as there is a risk of the patient inhaling more gas and getting anesthetised. Inhalation of the gas should be started a little before the desired analgesic effect is needed and should continue as long as analgesia is required.

2. **Halogenated agents**: Isoflurane, Desflurane, and Sevoflurane in sub-anaesthetic doses can be used for analgesia during labour. Sevoflurane has better acceptance and better pain relief at a concentration of 0.8%, although it is associated with more sedation. However, these agents are not commonly used in practice as they require specific vaporisers and because of other technical difficulties in their administration.

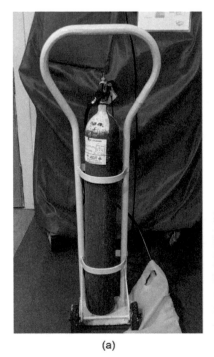
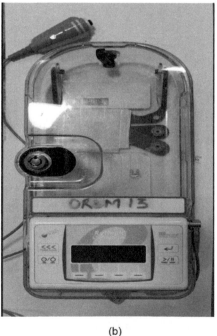

(a)   (b)

FIGURE 8.2   (a) Entonox cylinder. (b) Patient-controlled analgesia pump.

Parenteral Opioids

1. **Meperidine (Pethidine)**: Meperidine is a synthetic piperidine ester with opioid analgesic activity. It is one of the most commonly used opioids for labour and has been in independent use since the 1950s. The metabolism of meperidine gives rise to an active metabolite known as normeperidine. It has no major effects on the contractility of a gravid uterus but is contraindicated in severe pregnancy-induced hypertension as normeperidine has convulsant properties. Meperidine can cause sedation, confusional state, and respiratory depression in higher doses. Sometimes meperidine can cause desaturation, which is exacerbated when used together with Entonox.

   Meperidine crosses the placenta, and the fetal effects are largely based on the dosage and time of administration to the mother. As the respiratory centres in the neonate are not well developed, respiratory depression is seen more frequently in the neonate than in the mother. Normeperidine has increased half-life and adds to the neonatal effects of meperidine. The half-life of meperidine is 4 hours and that of normeperidine is 20 hours in the mother but 13 and 62 hours, respectively, in the baby. The use of meperidine in labour might make the baby sleep more and can have difficulties in the initiation of breastfeeding.

2. **Morphine**: Although morphine crosses the placenta rapidly, it does not cause a high morphine load in the fetus as maternal elimination is also fast. The dose used for maternal analgesia is a dose of 2–5 mg intravenous or 5–10 mg intramuscular and provides adequate pain relief to the mother. Morphine has a similar side effect profile as meperidine.

3. **Fentanyl**: Fentanyl is a lipid-soluble phenylpiperidine derivative. The main advantages of fentanyl are its rapid onset and short duration of action. Moreover, it does not give rise to any active metabolite.

4. **Remifentanil**: Remifentanil is a newer opioid analgesic drug with a very fast onset of action (1 minute) and an ultrashort duration of action also. Remifentanil does not accumulate in the body, and its context-sensitivity half-life is 4 minutes after a 4-hour infusion.

   Studies have shown remifentanil to provide satisfactory pain relief in labour. However, despite all these advantages, remifentanil can cause serious respiratory complications and needs monitoring to ensure safety.

NEURAXIAL TECHNIQUES (EPIDURAL AND COMBINED SPINAL EPIDURAL)

Neuraxial techniques are considered the present-day gold standard for labour analgesia. The two modalities used in neuraxial methods are epidural analgesia and combined spinal epidural analgesia.

INDICATIONS

1. **Maternal request**: This is the first and foremost indication of labour analgesia. In labour, in the absence of any medical contraindication, maternal request is sufficient for providing pain relief.

2. **Timing**: Earlier guidelines recommended that in nulliparous mothers, epidural analgesia should be delayed until the cervix dilates to 4–5 cm. Recent studies and trials have shown that epidural analgesia does not affect labour progress or mode of birth, even when started in the first stage of labour. Recommendations now state that no labouring woman wanting regional analgesia should be denied, irrespective of the stage of labour and cervical dilatation.

3. **Medical**: Neuraxial pain relief has beneficial effects on the fetus and mother. Maternal hyperventilation due to pain can cause resultant hypocarbia and reduction in uterine blood

flow and increase cardiac workload and stress at the time of contractions. All these reasons make neuraxial techniques specifically advantageous in parturients with pre-eclampsia and in those with cardiac, respiratory, and cerebrovascular comorbidities.

CONTRAINDICATIONS

Absolute contraindications to neuraxial labour techniques include a lack of consent, localised infection at the site, and increased intracranial tension.

Relative contraindications include sepsis, spinal cord lesions, thrombocytopenia, bleeding disorders, and patients on anticoagulant therapy. There is no standard cut-off value for platelet count in literature, below which neuraxial blockade is deemed unfit. Instead of the absolute value, the trend of change in platelet count along with platelet function is a better indicator.

EPIDURAL ANALGESIA

Epidural analgesia is the central component of labour pain management. After infiltration of the skin by a local anaesthetic agent, an epidural needle (Tuohy needle) and a loss of resistance to air/saline method is used to locate the epidural space. The depth of epidural space to the skin is noted using the markings on the Tuohy needle, and then the epidural catheter is threaded and fixed to the skin. For the analgesic block, a combination of local anaesthetic agent like bupivacaine or ropivacaine along with fentanyl is frequently used.

Maternal Positioning

Labour epidurals can be inserted in either a sitting or lateral decubitus position. However, in obese patients, it is difficult to palpate the midline in the lateral position, and in these patients sitting position is preferred.

Aseptic Technique

Meticulous aseptic technique should be followed during epidural insertion. Prior to the block, the skin should be thoroughly cleaned with chlorhexidine. Proper handwashing, along with the use of sterile clothing and gloves, is a must for the procedure.

Epidural Needles

The adult epidural needle is usually 16 G and 9 cm in length, with markings at 1 cm in length. The Tuohy needle is specially designed with a curved bevelled tip. This tip design helps in better perception as the needle tip pierces the various tissue structures and also helps in the threading of the catheter.

Loss of Resistance

The loss of resistance (LOR) technique is based on the fact that the various tissues and ligaments through which the needle progresses have different densities and resistance. Therefore, as the tip pierces the ligamentum flavum, there is an abrupt fall in the resistance felt, and this is known as loss of resistance. This technique can be used with fluid- or air-filled LOR syringes.

Epidural Catheters Fixation

When the epidural space is located with the LOR technique, the length of the needle inside is noted with the help of markings on the epidural needle. This is the distance of epidural space from the skin. Then the epidural catheter is threaded through the needle. If more catheter length is left inside the epidural space, then there are increased chances of kinking the catheter or the catheter entering an epidural vein. Similarly, if the length of the catheter kept inside is too short, then there is a higher risk of the catheter coming out. Usually, in practice, a length of 4–5 cm of the catheter is kept inside the epidural space.

Various types of sterile dressings and catheter locking devices have been used in the fixation of the catheter to skin, but there is no consensus on the optimal method.

Local Anaesthetic Agents

The three local anaesthetics commonly used in labour analgesia are bupivacaine, levobupivacaine, and ropivacaine.

Bupivacaine is a chiral mixture of levo- and dextro-isomers of bupivacaine. The onset is within 10 minutes. The effect peaks at 20 minutes, and the action lasts till around 160–220 minutes. If given intravenously or after toxic dose levels, bupivacaine is fatally cardiotoxic. It blocks potassium and sodium channels and can give rise to fatal arrhythmias.

Newer amide local anaesthetics are prepared as single enantiomers instead of chiral mixtures, and these have been shown to have a better safety profile and lesser cardiotoxicity. For example, levobupivacaine is the s-enantiomer of bupivacaine, with reduced cardiotoxic potential.

Ropivacaine has a similar chemical structure as bupivacaine, but its lipid solubility is less. It has a time of onset of 15–20 minutes, with a duration of 140–220 minutes.

As per the analgesic potency scale, levobupivacaine and ropivacaine have similar potency, while bupivacaine is more potent by about 40%. However, studies have shown that all three agents provide adequate analgesia and there is no appreciable effect on labour outcome.

Addition of Opioid

Fentanyl is a rapid-acting opioid analgesic and is used as an adjuvant to the local anaesthetic agent for the neuraxial blockade. It is commonly used in epidural preparations in a concentration of 2 mcg/ml and has a duration of action of 1 hour.

Commonly Used Concentrations for the Initiation of Labour Epidural

- Bupivacaine: 0.0625%–0.125%
- Levobupivacaine: 0.0625%–0.125%
- Ropivacaine: 0.06%–0.2%
- Fentanyl: 1–5 µg/mL

COMBINED SPINAL EPIDURAL (CSE)

In this method, initially, a subarachnoid block is given, after which the epidural catheter is threaded and fixed. The initial subarachnoid block takes care of the immediate pain relief, and then analgesia is maintained by top epidural ups. This method scores highly on the maternal satisfaction scale as the spinal block provides fast and immediate pain relief. As a result, CSE has become the standard technique of choice for labour analgesia in most institutions.

EPIDURAL OR CSE

Various studies and trials have failed to show any concrete authentication to propose one technique over another to initiate labour pain relief. The only slight advantage which makes the CSE technique desirable is the rapid pain relief which this method provides. Therefore, whether to initiate labour analgesia with CSE or just epidural depends on the institutional protocol, what the mother needs, fetal and neonatal safety, and the skills of the physician providing it.

MAINTENANCE

An ideal maintenance technique should provide continuous, uninterrupted, and safe analgesia and allow maternal ambulation. In addition, the incidence of breakthrough pain and the requirement of frequent top-ups should also be reduced.

After the initial loading dose, labour epidural dosing can be either through regular top-ups or continuous infusion. The first is the intermittent dosing method which consists of modalities such as regular manual top-ups and patient-controlled epidural analgesia (PCEA) (Figure 8.2b). In this, pain relief is provided at irregular intervals when the patient complains of pain. The second is the continuous method which prevents pain reoccurrence by providing continuous dosing of the medication and includes continuous epidural infusion (CEI), PCEA with basal infusion, and programmed intermittent epidural boluses (PIEB).

Most present institutional protocols follow the continuous epidural infusion method for maintenance, as this provides continuous analgesia compared to the irregular and sporadic pain relief by top-ups. The ongoing epidural process also avoids block regression and a painful waiting period.

COMPLICATIONS AND MANAGEMENT

1. **Hypotension**: Complete uterine displacement, intravenous fluids, and vasopressors.
2. **Post-dural puncture headache (PDPH)**: Bed rest, fluids, oral caffeine, non-steroidal anti-inflammatory drugs (NSAIDs), and epidural blood patch.
3. **Pruritus**: More common after intrathecal than epidural opioid administration. Opioid antagonists (e.g. naloxone) or partial agonist-antagonists (e.g. nalbuphine) are effective.
4. **Epidural hematoma**: Neurologic deficits are rarely seen in the obstetric population due to haematoma. Reassurance and conservative management usually resolve the deficit over time.
5. **Unexpected high block**: Communicate with the patient, avoid aortocaval compression, administer 100% oxygen, positive-pressure ventilation/intubate, and support maternal circulation with intravenous fluids and vasopressors.

CONCLUSION

The medical practice of labour analgesia has improved exponentially from the early days of ether and chloroform to the present-day practice, which is evidence-based medicine of labour pain management. Experiencing pain that is unbearable by the parturient is no longer considered acceptable. A request for analgesia during this period should not be deprived unless contraindication due to medical reason exists.

The introduction of newer techniques like combined spinal epidurals, low-dose epidurals facilitating ambulation, pharmacological advances like remifentanil for patient-controlled intravenous analgesia, and newer local anaesthetics like ropivacaine and levobupivacaine all have revolutionised the practice of pain management in labour. In addition, technological advances like the use of ultrasound to localise epidural space under challenging cases and novel drug delivery modalities such as PCEA pumps and computer-integrated drug delivery pumps have made it possible to individualise the treatment required and safety along with maternal satisfaction.

Recent randomised controlled trials and studies have shown that the association of epidurals with increased caesarean section and long-term backache remains only a myth. Studies have also shown that the newer, low-dose regimes do not have a statistically significant impact on the duration of labour and breastfeeding. These reduce the instrumental delivery rates, thus improving maternal and fetal safety.

An appropriate institution-based consent along with an explanation of risk and consequences should be available before providing the modality for analgesia. In addition, relevant education, knowledge, and competence should be in place by the team identified for delivering the peripartum obstetric analgesia care.

A quote by Moir aptly concludes this chapter:

> The delivery of the infant into the arms of a conscious and pain-free mother is one of the most exciting and rewarding moments in medicine.

9 Intrapartum Fetal Surveillance

Anish Keepanasseril
Jawaharlal Institute of Postgraduate Medical
Education and Research (JIPMER)

FETAL PHYSIOLOGY IN INTERPRETATION OF THE CARDIOTOCOGRAPHY FINDINGS

All living beings have an in-built mechanism to compensate for the stress from exposure to hypoxia, prioritising the blood supply to the myocardium (the physiologic pump) as its failure will result in decreased tissue perfusion in other organs. Coronary arteries are the first branch, from the root of the aorta (having maximum oxygenation) to supply myocardium, followed by the carotids from the arch of the aorta that supplies the brain. When exposed to hypoxic stress, the initial physiologic response is an increase in the respiratory rate. An increase follows this in the depth of respiration, which maintains the positive energy balance to the myocardium to maintain aerobic metabolism.

Catecholamine release in response to stress helps by increasing the heart rate and force of contraction of the myocardium as well as by diverting blood from the less important circulation (such as skin and gut) by triggering peripheral vasoconstriction. The vasoconstriction also increases the blood pressure, which helps to increase the force with which blood is delivered to central organs. The ability to respond to hypoxic stress seems to be greater with the fetus than the adults because of the increased amount of haemoglobin which has a higher oxygen affinity.

Unlike adults, the fetus cannot protect the myocardium from hypoxic injury by increasing the rate and depth of respiration. As the stroke volume cannot be increased, the increase in cardiac output in the fetus is mainly by the increase in the heart rate. This redistribution of fetal circulation and the increase in cardiac output to avoid the injury from hypoxia of the central organ may result in rapid myocardial hypoxia and acidosis, resulting in bradycardia. Hypoxia thus can result in acidosis and low intracellular pH, which can compromise cellular function and cell death. Fetuses respond by reducing the activity and reducing the heart rate leading to less demand of oxygen by myocardial fibres. The reduced rate will in turn increase oxygenation by increasing the diastolic filling of the coronary circulation. Once the oxygenation is restored, the fetus will recover the heart rate to baseline or even higher, due to the catecholamine release during hypoxic stress.[1]

Most of the fetuses with low Apgar score and even metabolic acidosis recover quickly without any short- or long-term complications. In the short term, it can lead to hypoxic ischaemic encephalopathy (HIE). This condition is categorised into three grades as per the classification proposed by Sarnat and Sarnat in 1976.[2] The development of neonatal seizures and coma with the documentation of the metabolic acidosis in the umbilical cord early after birth suggests the severity of neurological dysfunction in the newborn. It can also lead to the involvement of cardiovascular, gastrointestinal, haematological, renal, or even pulmonary systems. This can lead to long-term sequelae, i.e. cerebral palsy. Hypoxic injury during birth is attributed to 20%–30% of cases of cerebral palsy. Intrapartum surveillance can help for the early identification of fetuses with hypoxia, but care should be taken that it does not lead to unnecessary intervention such as caesarean section or instrumental delivery.[3]

DOI: 10.1201/9781003034360-9

RISK FACTORS OF INCREASED INTRAPARTUM FETAL COMPROMISE[3]

Various factors are recognised to increase the risk of fetal compromise during labour which may be identified in the antenatal or intrapartum period. The factors which are associated with the reduction in fetal reserve or affect the transport of oxygen in fetoplacental circulation can increase the risk of fetal compromise during labour. The antenatal risk factors include fetal growth restriction, oligo-hydramnios, antepartum haemorrhage, uterine scar, preeclampsia, previous bad obstetric history, abnormal fetal Doppler indices, multiple pregnancies, breech presentation, and prolonged pregnancy. The intrapartum risk factors include induction or augmentation of labour, maternal pyrexia during labour, blood or meconium-stained liquor, preterm labour, tachysystole, uterine hypertonus, and epidural analgesia.

METHODS OF INTRAPARTUM SURVEILLANCE

The commonly used methods for intrapartum surveillance include intermittent auscultation using a stethoscope, handheld Doppler, and electronic fetal heart monitoring with cardiotocography (CTG). Newer techniques are mostly used as adjunctive to the use of CTG. With each method offering some advantages and having some disadvantages, the use of methods should be tailored to the individual patient scenario and availability in a particular institution.

INTERMITTENT AUSCULTATION[4]

This refers to listening for short periods, without visualising the pattern, to the fetal heart rates using a stethoscope or a handheld Doppler device. After explaining the procedure to the pregnant woman, assessment of the fetal position by abdominal palpation to identify the position of the fetal back for placement of the stethoscope or the Doppler probe to hear the fetal heart rate is performed. Simultaneous assessment of the maternal pulse is helpful to reassure and confirm the fetal heart rate, and a hand over the uterine fundus determine the timing of contraction as well the fetal movements (Figure 9.1 and Table 9.1).

It is recommended to use a large (at least 7″) battery-powered clock with a quartz movement. One must listen for one full minute while counting in 5-second increments (i.e. 12 samplings per 60 seconds). Every 5 seconds, the count may vary from 10 to 14. It is possible with practice to listen to heart rate, rhythm, and variability (or lack of variability). Thus, intermittent auscultation should be intelligent and structured.

Performing intermittent auscultation ensures frequent contact between the women in labour and the monitoring personnel. This can help to provide social and clinical support. A provider can also check other parameters such as temperature, breathing pattern, and maternal contractions, in various positions comfortable to the labouring women, which can help assess labour progress. It is a method that is easily available and sustainable and can be used easily in limited-resource settings. However, this method poses the challenge of a longer learning curve to distinguish accelerations or decelerations, and it is difficult to identify the subtle changes even for an expert. Since there are no independent records available and subjectively heard only by the personnel auscultating, there may be uncertainty during case reviews and for legal issues unless the handheld Doppler method is used.

CARDIOTOCOGRAPHY[5–7]

The introduction of cardiotocography in the 1970s was one of the most important landmarks in the evolution of intrapartum fetal monitoring. The meta-analysis and the systematic reviews do not show any significant reduction in the major outcomes such as perinatal mortality or long-term neurological morbidity (cerebral palsy). However, its use is still advocated by most professional bodies for surveillance during labour and delivery. It should not be regarded as a substitute for

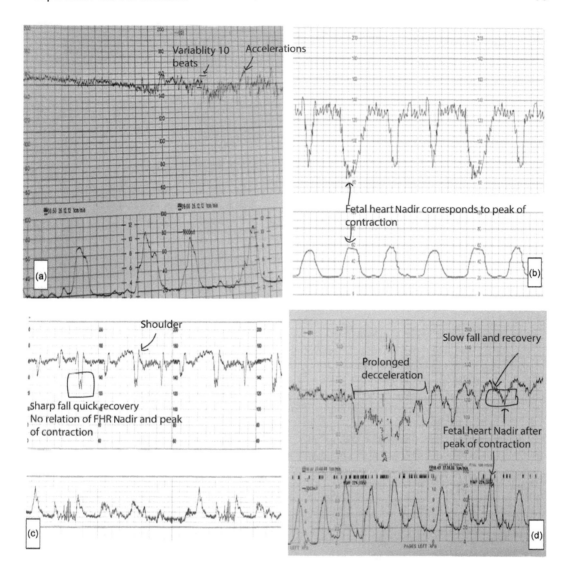

FIGURE 9.1 (a) Normal pattern. (b) Early deceleration. (c) Variable deceleration. (d) Late deceleration and a short segment of prolonged bradycardia.

good clinical judgement and observation nor as an excuse to leave a labouring mother alone. It is also used to assess the risk of major perinatal events in labour at the time of admission (admission CTG) even though there is a lack of evidence to continue such practice. In women with high-risk factors either before or during labour or when they are found to have an abnormality on intermittent auscultation, continuous CTG is advocated as the preferred method of monitoring the fetus in labour.

As the supine hypotension can occur with a maternal supine recumbent position, it is preferable to perform CTG in lateral, half sitting, or even upright positions. In most centres, wired sensors are used for acquiring the signals. However, in high-income countries, it is being switched over to wireless telemetric sensors, which allow free maternal movement during the acquisition of signals. Paper speed or the horizontal scale is usually set at 1 cm/minute, which allows sufficient details for clinical analysis with the advantage of reduced tracing length. The vertical scale may differ based on the paper and the setting, with most varying between 20 and 30 bpm/cm. Continuous external

TABLE 9.1

Checklist for Intermittent Auscultation

Parameter	Evaluation/Assessment
FHR	Duration: For at least 60 seconds, for three contractions if the FHR is not always in the normal range (110–160 bpm)
	Timing: During and at least 30 seconds after a contraction
	Interval:
	First stage: Every 15 minutes in the active phase
	Second stage: Every 5 minutes
	Document: Baseline as single count and presence of any acceleration or decelerations
Uterine contraction	Before and during FHR auscultation to detect the time interval between two contractions (which should be more than 2 minutes)

TABLE 9.2

Features of a Normal CTG

Term	Definition
Baseline	Refers to the mean level of the fetal heart rate. It should be interpreted from a segment that is stable without oscillations, accelerations and decelerations, and contractions. It is typically determined over 5 or 10 minutes and expressed in bpm. Preterm fetuses tend to have values towards the upper end of this range. A progressive rise in the baseline is important as well as the absolute values
Variability	The minor fluctuations around the baseline FHR. It is assessed by estimating the difference in beats per minute between the highest peak and lowest trough of fluctuation in 1-minute segments of the trace between contractions
Acceleration	Abrupt increases in FHR of 15 bpm or more above the baseline and lasting 15 seconds, but less than 10 minutes. Accelerations in the preterm fetus may be of lesser amplitude and shorter duration. The significance of no accelerations on an otherwise normal CTG is unclear
Deceleration	Transient decreases of the FHR below the baseline lasting at least 15 seconds
Early	Uniform, a repetitive decrease of FHR with slow onset early in the contraction and slow return to baseline by the end of the contraction. It has normal variability and coincides with the contractions; it is believed to be caused by fetal head compression
Late	Uniform, repetitive decreasing of FHR with, usually, slow onset mid to end of the contraction. Nadir more than 20 seconds after the peak of the contraction and ending after the contraction. In the presence of a non-accelerative trace with baseline variability <5 bpm, the definition would include decelerations of <15 bpm. These are indicative of chemoreceptor-induced hypoxia
Variable	Repetitive or intermittent decreasing of FHR with rapid onset and recovery. Time relationships with the contraction cycle may be variable but most commonly occur simultaneously with contractions. The most common type observed in labour is due to bara-receptor-mediated response as in umbilical cord occlusion
Prolonged	Fall in the baseline fetal heart rate for more than 90 seconds and up to 5 minutes. It indicates hypoxemia and is mediated through chemoreceptor-mediated response. They are frequently associated with fetal hypoxia or acidaemia
Tachysystole	Excessive frequency of contraction is defined as the occurrence of more than five contractions in 10 minutes in two successive periods of observation

fetal heart rate (FHR) monitoring with dual-channel monitors that allow simultaneous monitoring of both the fetuses during labour is advisable to avoid duplicate monitoring of the same twin.

CTG analysis is started with the evaluation of basic features followed by overall classification. Basic features include baseline, variability, accelerations, decelerations, and contractions.

Features of a normal CTG: Their criteria or evaluation and assessment with their abnormal values are shown in Table 9.2.

The traces in labour need to be evaluated in these basic features and classified into three categories: normal, suspicious, and pathological as suggested by the FIGO Intrapartum Expert Consensus panel. Further more, due to changes during labour, it advisable to re-evaluate the tracing every 30 minutes or earlier as the clinical situation warrants (Table 9.3).

Recently, with a better understanding of the fetal physiological response to hypoxia, the categorisation of the tracing based on the morphological classification of the deceleration is being reconsidered.

Based on the rapidity of the onset and the physiologic response, *hypoxia is classified into four types*[7]:

Acute Hypoxia

It presents with prolonged deceleration with a sudden drop in baseline to FHR < 80 bpm and persisting for more than 3 minutes. This can lead to rapid onset fetal metabolic acidosis. This usually occurs after intrapartum events such as abruptio placentae, umbilical cord prolapse, or uterine rupture, and the *pH decreases at a rate of >0.01 per minute*. If bradycardia does not recover, then we should follow the 3–6–9–12 minute rule. It recommends correcting the iatrogenic factor by 6 minutes, transferring the woman to the operation theatre by 9 minutes, commencing delivery by 12 minutes, and delivering within 15 minutes from the onset of deceleration if it doesn't recover.

Subacute Hypoxia

It presents with FHR remaining for <30 seconds on a stable baseline and decelerates for more than 90 seconds. The fetus spends more time with a heart rate that is decelerating and only one-third of

---

TABLE 9.3

Cardiotocography Classification Criteria, Interpretation, and Recommended Management[a] (as per FIGO Intrapartum Fetal Monitoring Expert Consensus Panel)[5]

	Normal	Suspicious	Pathological
Baseline	110–160 bpm	Lacking at least one characteristic of normality but with no pathological features	<100 bpm
Variability	5–25 bpm	Lacking at least one characteristic of normality but with no pathological features	Reduced variability, increased variability, or sinusoidal pattern
Decelerations	No repetitive decelerations[b]	Lacking at least one characteristic of normality but with no pathological features	Repetitive late or prolonged decelerations during >30 or 20 minutes if reduced variability, or one prolonged deceleration with >5 minutes
Interpretation	Fetus with no hypoxia/acidosis	Fetus with a low probability of having hypoxia/acidosis	Fetus with a high probability of having hypoxia/acidosis
Clinical management	No intervention necessary to improve fetal oxygenation state	Action to correct reversible causes if identified, close monitoring, or additional methods to evaluate fetal oxygenation	Immediate action to correct reversible causes, additional methods to evaluate fetal oxygenation, or if this is not possible, expedite delivery. In acute situations (cord prolapse, uterine rupture, or placental abruption), immediate delivery should be accomplished

[a] The presence of accelerations denotes a fetus that does not have hypoxia/acidosis, but their absence during labour is of uncertain significance.

[b] Decelerations are repetitive when they are associated with more than 50% of uterine contractions.

the time at baseline to exchange gases and to protect its brain. It can lead to the development of fetal acidosis with a drop in *pH at a rate of 0.01 per 2–3 minutes*. Once it happens, rule out the occurrence of uterine hyperstimulation, and in case it occurs in the second stage, the mother needs to stop pushing, which will help for fetal oxygenation to recover.

Gradually Evolving Hypoxia

The fetus has sufficient time to mobilise its reserve to compensate, starting with deceleration followed by loss of accelerations and release of catecholamines. The release of catecholamine leads to an increase in baseline FHR, which helps redistribute blood to vital organs and aid in the oxygenation of the circulation across the placenta. In case the compensation fails, decompensation sets in with a decrease in perfusion to the brain and loss of variability. It can lead to a reduction of oxygenation of the myocardium with resultant acidosis, which can be seen as instability of FHR baseline ending in stepladder pattern changes resulting in death.

Chronic Hypoxia

Chronic uteroplacental insufficiency causes pathological changes and results in a reduction in fetal reserve to compensate the hypoxia. The compensatory changes include an increase in baseline FHR, chemo-receptor-mediated decelerations (shallow deceleration with late recovery), and evidence of decompensation (loss of baseline variability). These fetuses might decompensate early with the onset of uterine contractions leading to progressive reduction in the FHR, indicating a need for early delivery. If the fetuses at 40 weeks present with baseline FHR > 150 bpm, a possibility of chronic hypoxia needs to be ruled out.

A method to interpret and manage based on the physiologic evaluation for CTG interpretation can be performed following the steps using **8 C's approach.**[8]

- **Step 1**: Clinical picture
  - Check the gestational age.
  - Assess the clinical picture to rule out any iatrogenic effect of medications administered, chorioamnionitis, meconium staining of liquor, presence of uterine scar, fetal malformations, intrapartum bleeding, and uterine hyperstimulation.
  - Review previous CTG traces if any
- **Step 2**: Cumulative uterine activity
  - It is the sum of frequency and duration of contraction in 10 minutes, assess whether there is an inter-contraction interval of 90 seconds which allows adequate oxygenation to the fetus.
- **Step 3**: Cycling of FHR
  - It is a sign of fetal well-being, which indicates alternate periods of activity and quiescence. The presence of accelerations suggests a healthy somatic nervous system.
  - The absence of cycling may occur in hypoxia, fetal infections including encephalitis, and intrauterine fetal stroke.
- **Step 4**: Central organ oxygenation
  - It is determined by the assessment of baseline FHR and variability.
  - Baseline FHR: Function of the myocardium due to electrical activity of SA node, modified by the autonomic nervous system and medications/catecholamine
  - Baseline variability reflects the status of the autonomic nervous system.
  - Loss of baseline variability and unstable baseline suggest the presence of central hypoxia, which indicates the need for urgent intervention to improve uteroplacental circulation/ delivery if the measures are ineffective.
- **Step 5**: Catecholamine surge
  - In fetuses exposed to slowly evolving hypoxia, the release of catecholamines leads to a slow and progressive increase in baseline FHR over several hours. Suppose the

correction of factors such as stopping/reducing oxytocin or changing maternal position did not improve the oxygenation. In that case, it will lead to decompensation (loss of baseline variability), leading to terminal fetal bradycardia secondary to myocardial hypoxia and acidosis.

- **Step 6**: Chemo- or baroreceptor decelerations
  - Deceleration indicates hypoxia from head compression, umbilical cord compression, and uteroplacental insufficiency. Chemoreceptor-mediated response is seen as a slow recovery to baseline FHR, whereas the baroreceptor-mediated response will have a sharp fall and an instantaneous recovery to the baseline. A fetal response can be noted in between the decelerations (a stable baseline with reassuring variability indicate good oxygenation of the central nervous system and a rise in baseline suggest an ongoing catecholamine surge).
- **Step 7**: Cascade
  - With the need for additional tests and the intervention to confirm or exclude the intrapartum hypoxia, one should understand the clinical picture and the type of the hypoxia and the fetal response to the hypoxic stress. Missing out on this response can lead to cascading events leading to loss or unnecessary interventions.
- **Step 8**: Consider the next change in the CTG trace.
  - In the event of the progress of hypoxia, first, the decelerations appear, which will become wider and deeper with time. It follows the absence of acceleration to conserve the energy that precedes the catecholamine surge, leading to rising baseline, and finally leading to unstable baseline and terminal bradycardia. The speed and the intensity of the progression depend on the physiological reserve of the fetus.

INTRAUTERINE RESUSCITATION

The concept of intrauterine resuscitation is changing. The routine convention of intravenous fluid infusion, oxygen by mask, is necessary only when the blood pressure is low or the oxygen saturation is reduced. Empirical use of the two may not necessarily help. More important is to address the underlying cause. When faced with an abnormal pattern of CTG during monitoring, causes can be identified, and alleviating them will lead to the improvement of fetal oxygenation leading to recovery to a normal reactive trace in most of the situations. Most commonly, excessive uterine activity is the cause of fetal hypoxia, which can be detected by palpation and assessing strength, frequency, duration, and the tone between the contractions. In most cases, it can be reversed by stopping the oxytocin infusion, removing prostaglandins administered, if possible, and using tocolysis with beta-mimetics such as terbutaline. When it happens during the second stage, maternal pushing efforts may be asked to be stopped to see whether the trace improves, in the absence of which delivery needs to be expedited. Changing maternal position can lead to a reduction of (i) supine hypotension, (ii) transient cord compressions, and also (iii) excessive uterine activity from stimulation of the sacral plexus. Administration of fluid boluses can improve the sudden maternal hypotension, especially following spinal or epidural analgesia.

The widely used practices such as (i) hydration with intravenous fluid in a normotensive woman and (ii) oxygenation in an otherwise well-oxygenated mother are not supported by evidence from the literature and may even be harmful. A good and timely clinical assessment for the cause of the abnormal pattern to judge its reversibility can determine the timing as well the mode of delivery to avoid the use of unnecessary obstetric interventions

ADJUNCTIVE TECHNOLOGIES FOR INTRAPARTUM MONITORING[7,9]

Even though the sensitivity of the CTG is high, the low specificity for predicting fetal hypoxia/acidosis can lead to increased chances of unnecessary interventions. In conditions other than a reassuring CTG where the state of fetal oxygenation can be considered normal, the use of adjunctive methods can help to assess the oxygenation. Over the last few decades, these methods include fetal blood sampling, continuous pH and lactate monitoring, fetal stimulation, pulse oximetry, and ST wave analysis (STAN). A brief description of the methods as well the concepts guiding its usage in intrapartum monitoring is described below. Among these methods, continuous pH monitoring and fetal pulse oximetry are no longer in use due to the technical challenges and risk of complications.

FETAL SCALP STIMULATION

It involves the stimulation of the fetal scalp by either rubbing with a finger during an examination or using forceps to clasp the fetal skin or externally with vibroacoustic stimulation to the mother's abdomen. It is mainly used in a situation where the variability is reduced in CTG to differentiate between quiescent sleep state and hypoxia/acidosis. Acceleration and increase in variability in sleep following stimulation with normalisation of the pattern after stimulation are considered reassuring, and this finding is shown to have a good negative predictive value in excluding hypoxia.

FETAL BLOOD SAMPLING (FBS)

A good correlation has been reported between the pH and lactate obtained from the fetal scalp with that of the umbilical vein and artery. Therefore, FBS from the scalp is used as a method to assess fetal hypoxemia in cases with suspicious and pathological CTG. However, in the cases of a severe fetal distress and acute event such as abruption, it's advisable to deliver by caesarean section without delay for getting an FBS done. The blood collected in the heparin-coated capillary tube from the scalp can fail to obtain information regarding the blood gases in 10% and lactate in nearly 2%. A report of pH < 7.2 or the lactate levels > 4.8 mmoL/L indicates an urgent action for normalisation of CTG pattern or rapid delivery. Normal lactate levels suggest the absence of hypoxia or acidosis when performed in the last hour of labour. Various algorithms are followed by professional bodies in developed nations for reducing unnecessary intervention based only on CTG findings. As the changes during labour are dynamic, information obtained from the FBS can be quickly outlived, suggesting the need for repetition of the sampling. This may be considered as the main limitation. It is difficult to obtain a sample in early labour with lower cervical dilatation and it also carries a small risk of bleeding and infection.

FETAL ELECTROCARDIOGRAPHY (STAN REPORTING)

It involves the combination of standard CTG interpretation with concurrent analysis of the fetal electrocardiogram. During hypoxia, there is an increase in the height of the T wave, causing ST depression and inversion of the T wave. In the STAN software, the average waveform of the fetal ECG signal over 30 heartbeats is assessed for the changes in the ST segment and T wave, which is signalled as alerts or the STAN events. First, the CTG trace is interpreted, and the STAN events are looked for abnormalities. The primary limitation is that it cannot help in the situation where the fetus is already hypoxic at the first reading, as it looks for the change in the fetal ECG compared to the baseline at the start of the monitoring. *Cochrane Review* (2015) reported moderate evidence in the reduction of the fetal scalp blood sampling and fewer instrumental or operative deliveries.

INTRAPARTUM ULTRASOUND

Recently, ultrasound is gaining more popularity for objective assessment of the fetal head station and position, which could help early identification of delayed labour or arrest of labour and aid in the operative vaginal delivery safely. It helps in correctly diagnosing the fetal position and ruling out asynclitism in the presence of caput before contemplating assisted vaginal birth.

REFERENCES

1. Heuser CC. Physiology of Fetal Heart Rate Monitoring. *Clin Obstet Gynecol* 2020; **63**(3): 607–615.
2. Sarnat HB, Sarnat MS. Neonatal encephalopathy following fetal distress. A clinical and electroencephalographic study. *Arch Neurol* 1976; **33**(10): 696–705.
3. Ayres-de-Campos D, Arulkumaran S, Panel FIFMEC. FIGO consensus guidelines on intrapartum fetal monitoring: Physiology of fetal oxygenation and the main goals of intrapartum fetal monitoring. *Int J Gynaecol Obstet* 2015; **131**(1): 5–8.
4. Lewis D, Downe S, Panel FIFMEC. FIGO consensus guidelines on intrapartum fetal monitoring: Intermittent auscultation. *Int J Gynaecol Obstet* 2015; **131**(1): 9–12.
5. Ayres-de-Campos D, Spong CY, Chandraharan E, Panel FIFMEC. FIGO consensus guidelines on intrapartum fetal monitoring: Cardiotocography. *Int J Gynaecol Obstet* 2015; **131**(1): 13–24.
6. Santo S, Ayres-de-Campos D, Costa-Santos C, et al. Agreement and accuracy using the FIGO, ACOG, and NICE cardiotocography interpretation guidelines. *Acta Obstet Gynecol Scand* 2017; **96**(2): 166–175.
7. Pinas A, Chandraharan E. Continuous cardiotocography during labour: Analysis, classification, and management. *Best practice & research Clinical obstetrics & gynaecology* 2016; **30**: 33–47.
8. Intrapartum Fetal Monitoring Guideline - Physiological CTG. 2018. https://physiological-ctg.com/guideline.html (accessed 05th May 2021).
9. Visser GH, Ayres-de-Campos D, Panel FIFMEC. FIGO consensus guidelines on intrapartum fetal monitoring: Adjunctive technologies. *Int J Gynaecol Obstet* 2015; **131**(1): 25–29.

10 Understanding the Warning Signal of the Uterus and the Fetus

Gowri Dorairajan
Jawaharlal Institute of Postgraduate Medical
Education and Research (JIPMER)

When labour does not proceed as per the timelines mentioned in Chapter 4, it is perceived as abnormal. There are various reasons for labour progress becoming abnormal. Quite a few of these situations can be anticipated. It is rewarding to identify the underlying risk factors that forewarn problems during labour. About 10%–15% of labour can become abnormal.

PREDISPOSING FACTORS

Following are a few predisposing factors.

Advanced maternal age: The tissues become less elastic with advancing age. The pelvic tissue resistance is high. The joints are likely to be less pliable. All this could result in abnormal delay and dystocia in labour.

Obesity: It is more often associated with PROM, chorioamnionitis, unfavourable cervix, and longer labour [1]. Obesity changes the fetal placental weight ratio. The adipose tissue alters the oestrogen–progesterone ratio at term, making the myometrium less sensitive to prostaglandin E2. The adipokines alter the myometrial contraction synchronization, and the gap junction and uterine connexin-43 are altered in obesity [2].

Malposition: Fetus in posterior occipital position present with deflexed head. Occipitoposterior positions are known to be associated with prolonged labour due to the time taken for the long rotation. The ill-fitting head results in an elongated bag of membranes that can rupture prematurely. This further drains the liquor and prolongs labour even more.

Big baby: Big babies can prolong labour. The bigger head takes time to undergo moulding to negotiate the pelvic diameters. The labour gets prolonged, especially after reaching the transition phase.

Malformations: Cephalic presentation with hydrocephalous needs vigilance for disproportion. An intervention by tapping of the head to reduce the engaging diameters may be required when there is dystocia. This should be done after counselling and weighing the prognosis of the condition and salvageability of the fetus. Hydrocephalous presenting as breech needs vigilance in the second stage for tapping through the foramen magnum to aid in the delivery of the large head. Other malformations such as sacrococcygeal teratoma, soft tissue problems such as massive fetal ascites, abdominal tumours, and conjoined twins can also cause serious dystocia late in labour.

Short stature: This warns about the possible inadequate pelvis. The height cut-off varies from population to population. A height of 140 cm and less has an absolute risk of caesarean of 30% [3]. A cut-off of 145 cm was found to be associated with higher odds (OR 2.4) of caesarean section due to dystocia [4]. So, the height of the women should alert us. A careful, thorough assessment of the

DOI: 10.1201/9781003034360-10

fetal position, fetal weight, and pelvic architecture should be done for these women. Increased vigilance during labour is necessary for diagnosing dystocia in such situations.

Polyhydramnios: Excessive distension of the uterus not only makes the uterine contraction incoordinate but also ineffective. The inability of the presenting part to fix properly further prolongs labour and delays cervical dilation.

Post-term pregnancy: Post-term pregnancies are more likely to have unfavourable cervix and induction of labour. A post-term head has a limited capacity to mould due to reduced elasticity. All this results in labour dystocia and higher chances of caesarean section.

Chorioamnionitis: Infection sets in certain changes in the myometrium. This makes the contractions ineffective and can prolong labour and even predispose to atonic postpartum haemorrhage. Prolonged labour, on the other hand, can cause chorioamnionitis and further tardy the labour progress.

Multiple gestations: Overdistension of the uterus can cause prolonged labour due to dysfunctional contractions.

Maternal stress response: The catecholamines secreted due to maternal stress inhibit the uterine contractions. Fear of childbirth increases the stress response. It is very important to assess the anxiety and fear levels of the women about childbirth. Antenatal counselling and teaching relaxation and breathing exercise help mentally prepare them and reduce labour stress levels [3].

Malformations of the uterus: Malformations of the uterus, especially the unicornuate uterus, are likely to be associated with dysfunctional uterine contractions.

Malpresentations: Among the cephalic presentation, if the brow is the presenting part or the head is extremely deflexed resulting in median presentation, then the engaging diameters of the fetal head are larger. This results in difficult negotiation and abnormal labour in the form of protraction or arrest of labour. Compound presentation such as head with the hand can also complicate and prevent normal progress of labour. Of course, malpresentation such as a transverse lie can be an obvious cause of abnormal labour.

Obstruction: Obstruction due to myomas or tumours in the pelvis can also be a rare cause for abnormal labour.

Cervical factors such as stenosis, prolapse, and previous surgeries can also predispose to abnormal labour. The scarred tissue of the cervix may fail to dilate despite good contractions.

Certain features should alert us about the likelihood of predisposing factors. These *alerting factors* are:

a. **Lack of spontaneous labour**: If nature has not put a woman into labour even after she has crossed the expected date of delivery by more than a week and the Bishop score remains less than 6, then it is a matter of concern. Malpositions and cephalometric disproportion should be ruled out by careful reassessment.

b. **Term premature rupture of membranes with poor Bishop Score**: This should draw attention towards malposition. The elongated bag of membranes tends to rupture prematurely.

c. **Need for augmentation of labour**: Need for oxytocin in women after achieving the spontaneous active phase is an alert. One must watch for other predisposing factors such as malposition and cephalopelvic disproportion. Secondary inertia of the uterus is sometimes a protective phenomenon against difficult operative delivery in the second stage.

d. **Dysfunctional labour**: Occurrence of incoordinate contractions, spastic lower segment, etc. are indirect warning signs of some problems. Whether it is the cause or effect or a protective mechanism preventing labour from proceeding is not clear. This is an important signal given by the uterine muscles and needs to be perceived and interpreted correctly by obstetricians.

e. **Meconium-stained liquor**: Meconium-stained liquor in the absence of growth retardation or postdates is an alert. One must attempt to reassess carefully to rule out cephalopelvic disproportion. Any addition of hypoxia or asphyxia due to prolonged labour or disproportion can add to the morbidity due to meconium aspiration and can increase the risk of perinatal mortality.

f. **Deflexed head**: This implies a bigger diameter of the head will negotiate the maternal diameters and alert us to monitor labour progress carefully. It should also increase vigilance on fetal heart sounds as the nuchal cord is a distinct possibility. It also alerts us to look for malposition. Labour is likely to be prolonged in the presence of a deflexed head.

CLINICAL FEATURES AND IDENTIFICATION OF ABNORMAL LABOUR

Some subtle signs can start appearing even before a fully established abnormal labour and forewarn us about problems in an otherwise low-risk woman. These are

1. **Maternal tachycardia**: It is more often due to the inability to bear the pain. It may also be a manifestation of extreme anxiety of the woman. Tachycardia can also set in due to subtle infection or dehydration of prolonged labour.
2. **Maternal dehydration**: This can result due to excessive groaning due to dysfunctional labour and prolonged labour.
3. **Excessive backache**: Some women experience continued backache over and above the intermittent lower abdominal pain of uterine contractions. This warns about a possible posterior position. Such continued severe backache can cause immense discomfort, and the woman may find it difficult to lie down. She may assume the knee-chest position or on all four positions. Pain relief with epidural analgesia should be considered in such woman if parental opioids are not sufficient.
4. **Labour graph crosses the alert line**: If the woman achieved the active phase and thereafter the progress of dilation is tardy, it requires reassessment, corrective measures, and diligent watch on progress.
5. **Need for augmentation**: The need for augmentation due to secondary inertia after spontaneously achieving the active phase of labour forewarns about occult cephalopelvic disproportion. Continued vigilance is necessary
6. **Dysfunctional uterine contractions** (detailed in Chapter 11). Occurrence of spastic lower segment, secondary inertia after achieving active phase and also primary inertia or prolonged latent phase due to hypotonic contraction should alert us. We should reassess such cases carefully by repeat assessment for the position, type of pelvis, and manifest features of disproportion.
7. The repeated urge to pass urine and the **urinary bladder getting filled up** and becoming palpable in the abdomen indicates subtle disproportion and compression of the urethrovesical junction by the advancing head. In such cases, careful revaluation of the pelvis should be performed and a second opinion taken from seniors or colleagues.
8. **Premature bearing down**: This is also indicative of rectal pressure due to occipitoposterior position and can cause cervical caput formation and exhaust the woman. Recognizing this problem and giving adequate analgesia are necessary.

The following findings on digital examination signify abnormal labour:

A. *Tardy or arrested cervical dilation* or descent of head after having achieved active phase of labour despite good uterine contractions (180–200 Montevideo) for 4 hours. If the graph crosses the alert line, as mentioned above, it needs evaluation for cause and if the cervical dilation graph crosses the action line despite good uterine contractions of more than 4 hours, it is abnormal labour and needs the decision to terminate by caesarean section.
B. *Cervical lips becoming thick and hanging loose*: In the active phase of labour, if the cervix which was well effaced and applied to the presenting part becomes gradually and

progressively thicker and hanging loose, it indicates abnormal labour. This is a manifestation of reduced venous drainage of the cervix that is caught between the head and the pelvis due to the tight fit of the head in the pelvis. Sometimes thick anterior lip alone in the absence of other features can happen as the anterior lip of the cervix get caught between the advancing head and the pubic symphysis. This is less worrisome a finding, and the anterior lip can be pushed beyond the presenting part by the examining finger.

C. *Caput formation*: The formation of pelvic caput is an ominous sign indicating abnormal labour (detailed later in the chapter).

D. *Moulding*: Score more than or equal to 4/6 indicates significant moulding and confirms abnormal labour due to disproportion (detailed later in this chapter).

E. *Coning of the head*: A finding less described in textbooks. This is a finding when the parietal bones meeting at the sagittal suture are not at the same plane and start forming a cone as they meet at the sagittal suture. If this is observed above the brim, then it indicates serious disproportion. Sometimes, even though the major diameter is above the brim, the head will appear to be at a lower station due to coning. It is important to appreciate this finding in women on brim trial with tardy progress.

F. *Continued deflexion*: In the presence of protracted or arrested progress of labour, palpation of diamond-shaped bregma on digital pelvic examination signifies deflexed head (median presentation). This, along with caput or moulding, signifies abnormal labour.

G. *Failure to achieve the active phase of labour*: Sometimes despite good uterine contractions the cervix never opens to even 4 cm and fails to fulfil the definition of the active phase. Cervical dystocia needs to be kept in mind. One could extend the trial for a further time with vigilance. It is more likely to happen in women who have had previous operations in the cervix, uterine prolapse, Mullerian malformations, and following previous operative deliveries.

H. *Persistent asynclitism*: It is another finding signifying abnormal labour. Posterior asynclitism in a primigravida is a warning sign of abnormal labour.

MOULDING

Moulding is the overlapping of the skull bones at the sutures in an attempt to reduce the diameter of the skull. It is an important adjustment made by the fetus to negotiate the maternal pelvis. Moulding would occur in one suture with the expansion of the brain in the 90° direction.

It is graded as:
- 0 when the bones are apart
- + when the bones have come in close approximation
- ++ when the bones overlap at the suture, but it is reducible
- +++ when the overlap is not reducible.

Moulding can occur in any of the three sutures, i.e. sagittal, coronal, or lambdoid suture. There is a scoring system proposed by Stewart long back in 1977. Score 0 for no moulding; score 1 if the suture line is closed, but there is no overlapping; 2 for reducible; and 3 is given for irreducible overlapping. He proposed the moulding to be observed in the sagittal and lambdoid suture. So, based on the number of sutures involved, the score can vary from 0 to 6/6. Moulding more than 4/6 is an ominous and confirmed sign of disproportion between the head and the pelvis during labour. Another score was proposed by Shilotri and Panat in 1985. They proposed the same above score but to be observed in the three suture lines: coronal, sagittal, and lambdoid suture. They proposed the highest score of 9 and a score equal to or more than 7 has poor neonatal outcome. During the digital examination, one must attempt to feel for moulding in all the sutures and score it. Scoring makes the assessment objective and reduces the subjective variations in mentioning mild, moderate, or severe moulding.

The presence of moulding in the sagittal suture is an indirect signal that the fetus is trying to reduce its transverse diameter. This means that the maternal diameter that is housing the biparietal diameter (for example, the anteroposterior diameter of the brim in cases of occipitotransverse position) of the fetus is borderline or narrow.

So the suture line that has maximum moulding gives a clue to the inadequate maternal diameter. Moulding in the coronal or lambdoid suture (Figure 10.1a) signifies that the maternal diameter (for example, right oblique of the brim in case of left occipitoanterior position) housing the longitudinal diameter (suboccipitobregmatic diameter if well-flexed head) is narrow.

Coning of the head (Figure 10.1b): This is a less described finding. It refers to both the parietal bones forming a cone at sagittal suture instead of undergoing moulding. This condition denotes a more severe form of disproportion. If the pelvis is contracted and cannot allow this, the head may start coning, especially in brim contraction cases. More details of this condition are given in Chapter 11.

CAPUT SUCCIDENUM

It is oedema of the scalp due to impaired venous drainage (Figure 10.1c). Caput usually manifests after the cushioning effect of the forewater bag of membranes filled with amniotic fluid is ruptured. The swelling can cross midline and suture lines. It is oedema in the scalp and pitting can be observed on pressing. It is transient and recovers with time after childbirth. There are two types of caput.

A. **Cervical caput**: This occurs when the tight ring of the cervix impairs the venous drainage of the scalp distal to the tight ring formed by the cervix. Premature bearing down pushes the leading part of the head against a tight cervical ring predisposing it to its formation.

Relieving pain and discouraging premature bearing down during labour help to reduce cervical caput formation. Teaching relaxing exercises and encouraging deep breathing with labour pains during the antenatal period itself is important. It will reduce maternal stress syndrome. Birth companion and distractions in the form of music, etc. also help.

B. **Pelvic caput**: This is a large caput formation across the whole scalp wedged against the bony confines of the pelvis. If the fit of the head is extremely tight against the pelvis, then the venous drainage of the scalp distal to the pelvis is prevented. This is a sign of severe cephalopelvic disproportion. Pelvic caput can obliterate the perception of the sutures and may confuse the obstetrician about the position of the head. The other caution is that the enlarging and advancing caput can be misperceived as advancing descent of the head, and the station of the head will be perceived as falsely low, especially by the inexperienced obstetrician.

Assessing the correct station and position in the presence of a large caput is critically important before deciding to apply an instrument. Otherwise, the instrumental delivery is likely to fail and may cause trauma to the woman and asphyxia to the fetus.

Figure 10.1c also shows cephalhematoma and subgaleal bleed, which is described in Chapter 15.

SYNCLITISM AND ASYNCLITISM

Normally, the sagittal suture of the fetal head is set such as to occupy the centre of the maternal pelvis during labour. So on digital vaginal examination, both the parietal bones are felt equally, and the sagittal suture is in the centre of the pelvis.

Asynclitism refers to the deflection of the sagittal suture anteriorly or posteriorly so that one of the parietal bones occupies the centre of the pelvic field.

Asynclitism is a mechanism of labour of the platypelloid pelvis. In a flat pelvis, the anteroposterior diameter at the inlet is narrow or reniform, but the transverse diameter at the inlet is the largest.

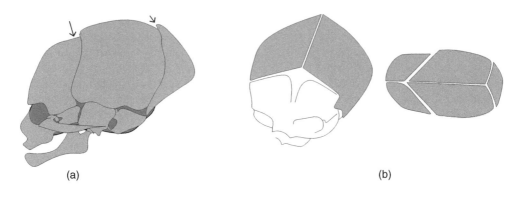

(a)   (b)

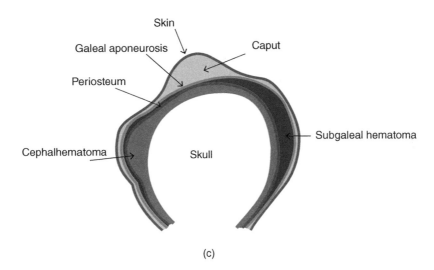

(c)

FIGURE 10.1 (a) Line diagram showing moulding in coronal and lambdoid sutures. (b) Line diagram showing coning of the head. (c) Line diagram showing caput succedaneum, cephalhematoma, and subgaleal hematoma.

The head presents as occipitotransverse position. The suboccipitobregmatic diameter of the fetus occupies the larger transverse diameter of the inlet of the pelvis. The biparietal diameter occupies the anteroposterior diameter of the inlet. Asynclitism shortens the transverse diameter to subparietoparietal diameter, which is about 8.4 cm. It is nearly 1 cm less than the biparietal diameter. A shorter transverse diameter of the head finds it easier to negotiate the narrow transverse diameter of the inlet of the pelvis.

Posterior asynclitism or posterior parietal presentation: The sagittal suture is deflected anteriorly under the pubic symphysis, and the posterior parietal bone is the presenting part. This is also called Liptzmans obliquity. This denotes that the anterior part of the forepelvis is narrow, and the wider posterior part is allowing the parietal bone to negotiate. Its persistence in a primigravida later in labour is a distinct sign of abnormality.

Anterior asynclitism or anterior parietal presentation: This denotes poor space posteriorly due to jutting forwards of sacral promontory and more available space anteriorly to allow the parietal bone to negotiate. This is also called Naegel's obliquity.

Asynclitism is a mechanism of labour in the flat pelvis in the early phase of labour, and once the head negotiates the brim and advances down, it gets corrected. Its persistence late in labour is a sign of abnormality and dictates the need to terminate by caesarean section. If the sagittal suture is in the anteroposterior diameter, then one can have right or left asynclitism. Sometimes it may be difficult to diagnose asynclitism on digital examination due to large caput formation. Intrapartum ultrasound [5,6] (a combination of transperineal and abdominal scan) is particularly helpful in such situations. In the presence of asynclitism, only one orbit will be visualized on the transverse section on the transabdominal scan. This is called a squint sign. The sunset of the thalamus and the cerebellar signs are other signs to diagnose asynclitism by ultrasound.

Observing and recording the above-mentioned signs help appropriate interpretation of the progress of labour. Every caregiver should observe and detail these findings, even if negative, after every internal examination. These findings help in deciding the mode of delivery.

REFERENCES

1. Hautakangas, T., Palomäki, O., Eidstø, K. et al. Impact of obesity and other risk factors on labor dystocia in term primiparous women: A case control study. *BMC Pregnancy Childbirth*. 2018;18, 304. doi: 10.1186/s12884-018-1938-3.
2. Carlson, N.S., Hernandez, T.L. & Hurt, K.J. Parturition dysfunction in obesity: Time to target the pathobiology. *Reprod Biol Endocrinol*. 2015;13, 135. doi: 10.1186/s12958-015-0129-6.
3. Lowe, N.K. A review of factors associated with dystocia and cesarean section in nulliparous women. *J Midwifery Women's Health*. 2007;52(3):216–228.
4. Toh-adam, R., Srisupundit, K., & Tongsong, T. Short stature as an independent risk factor for cephalopelvic disproportion in a country of relatively small-sized mothers. *Arch Gynecol Obstet*. 2012;285(6): 1513–1516. Published online 2011 Dec 21. doi: 10.1007/s00404-011-2168-3.
5. Malvasi, A., Tinelli, A. & Stark, M. Intrapartum sonography sign for occiput posterior asynclitism diagnosis. *J Matern Fetal Neonatal Med* 2011; 24: 553–554.
6. Malvasi, A., Stark, M., Ghi, T., Farine, D., Guido, M. & Tinelli, A. Intrapartum sonography for fetal head asynclitism and transverse position: Sonographic signs and comparison of diagnostic performance between transvaginal and digital examination. *J Matern Fetal Neonatal Med*. 2012;25(5):508–512. doi: 10.3109/14767058.2011.648234. Epub 2012 Feb 14.

11 Abnormal Uterine Contractions

Gowri Dorairajan
Jawaharlal Institute of Postgraduate Medical
Education and Research (JIPMER)

The uterus is the powerhouse for the completion of the fetal journey. Therefore, it is important to understand the language of the uterus during labour. The uterine contractions are the way the uterine myofibrils communicate. The contractions must proceed in a coordinated, synchronous, regular, and uniform way to generate adequate power to pull the cervix open and to push the fetus in the right direction along the curve of Carus to complete its journey from the pelvis to the outside world.

So, there is a polarity to the normal uterine contractions. These start at the fundus (pacemaker near the ostia) and spread uniformly all around and proceed downwards towards the lower segment. We learnt about the characteristics of a normal uterine contraction (Figure 11.1a) in Chapter 5.

CLASSIFICATION OF ABNORMAL UTERINE CONTRACTIONS

The abnormal uterine contractions (Figure 11.1b onwards) could be with

- Normal polarity
- Abnormal polarity

Normal polarity includes hypotonic contractions or primary inertia when the uterine contractions are not strong enough from the beginning. Secondary inertia can occur after an established active phase of labour due to certain reasons such as malposition and contracted pelvis. On the other end of the spectrum, we can have a situation of too strong a contraction in obstructed labour, as the uterus tries its level best to overcome the obstruction. Too strong a contraction can also cause precipitate labour. *Abnormal polarity* includes colicky uterus, spastic lower segment, tetanic uterus, and constriction ring.

The dysfunctional uterine contractions can manifest in various ways, as described below.

Prolonged latent phase: This is a condition where women experience uterine contractions that are strong enough to cause pain but do not improve and remain ineffective in bringing out a change in cervical dilation. It means there are inadequate or hypotonic contractions. The polarity is maintained. Usually, it does not exhaust the woman, but if active labour fails to establish, the woman becomes tired even before she goes into established labour. Therefore, the latent phase is the time from the onset of perceived painful uterine contractions till the beginning of the active phase of labour. This phase helps to soften and efface the cervix. This phase is likely to be more marked in those who had not undergone prelabour changes in the cervix. It is more likely also in those with occiput posterior position, those undergoing induction of labour, and those who develop premature rupture of membranes, polyhydramnios, and multiple gestations. Psychological factors such as anxiety and fear can also play a role. It can also be associated with injudicious use of sedatives and analgesics. Past dates and chorioamnionitis have also been found to be associated with prolonged latent phase in a multigravida.[1] Prolonged latent phase with the cervix opened to 1–2 cm is also a forerunner for difficult labour and occult cephalopelvic disproportion, emergency caesarean section, and adverse outcomes.[2,3]

DOI: 10.1201/9781003034360-11

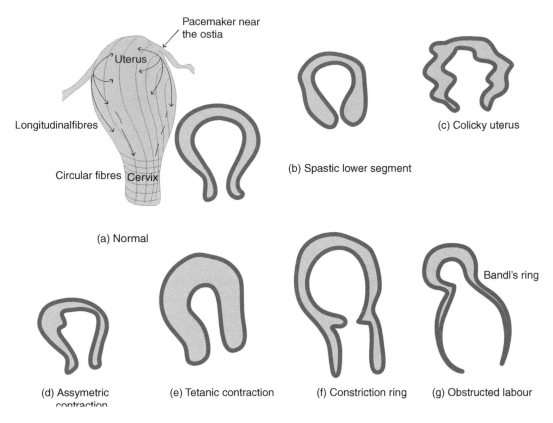

FIGURE 11.1 (a–g) Line diagram showing the pacemaker and normal uterine contraction and the various dysfunctional uterine contraction.

The treatment of choice is rest for a while and continued monitoring. Sedation helps to give temporary relief, but repeated sedation should be avoided. Peanut-shaped birthing balls are helpful for correcting the malpositions.[4] A warm bath, breathing deep and slow, keeping distracted with some work, and having a good diet and plenty of fluids also help in tiding over the painful but ineffective cramps of the latent phase. It may require augmentation with oxytocins in those where delivery needs to be expedited. Once again, close watch for features of disproportion and fetal heart rate monitoring is warranted. These women are more prone to develop retained placenta and postpartum bleeding due to atonicity.

Dysfunctional or incoordinate uterine contractions due to abnormal polarity: If the uterus loses polarity, then the pacemaker may become multiple or shift to an abnormal focus, and labour may become abnormal. These are described below.

TETANIC UTERINE CONTRACTIONS

In this condition, the uterus tends to go into a prolonged contraction involving the both the upper and lower segment. The basal tone becomes high, and the woman has exaggerated pain and is not comfortable even in between two contractions. Multiple diffuse pacemakers initiate this kind of generalised spasm. On abdominal examination, the uterus appears tense and tender and somewhat smaller. The fetal parts are not easily delineated, and the fetal heart sounds may appear muffled. With a close differential diagnosis of abruption, one tends to do artificial rupture of membranes to observe the colour of the liquor.

On vaginal examination, the cervix may appear thick and oedematous. A large caput or moulding would suggest underlying cephalopelvic disproportion. There could be malposition. In addition to these underlying factors, this condition can be caused by the overzealous use of oxytocin. The mother is exhausted very fast, and the foetus can manifest distress. Rupture uterus is unlikely. There is no differentiation in the upper and lower segment. In the absence of features of disproportion, the treatment lies in stopping oxytocin, giving sedation/epidural analgesia, and intravenous fluids to correct dehydration and ketosis and await for spontaneous correction. Antibiotics may be needed if the woman is in prolonged labour. One needs to exercise caution in restarting oxytocin for these patients, and restricting the oxytocin dose to much lesser than earlier would be prudent. The findings reported in case the women were delivered by caesarean section is that the lower segment is not well-formed because it is thick. This is ironic because the lower segment gets well-formed in labour. This condition can result in active retention of the fetus. Invariably, caesarean might be performed for fetal distress.

SPASTIC LOWER UTERINE SEGMENT

In this condition, the lower segment contraction predominates and tends to go into spasm. The woman gets an urge to pass urine repeatedly, is in constant pain, and has an urge to bear down prematurely. On abdominal examination, the pelvic grip will trigger more uterine contraction and pain. The woman may not allow the pelvic grip examination, though the uterus is relaxed, allowing other grips. The pelvis grip findings become obscured. On vaginal examination, the cervix appears thick and hanging loose, not well applied to the presenting part. Meconium-stained liquor may be manifested due to fetal compromise. Ruling out cepahlopelvic disproportion is important. Treatment is in the same lines as generalised tetanic contractions.

Asymmetric uterine contractions, colicky uterus, etc. are other manifestations of abnormal polarity.

In abnormal polarity, the women appear in constant discomfort and pain, but the labour does not progress as expected because the contractions are ineffective.

CONSTRICTION RING (SCHROEDER'S RING)

This is dysfunctional labour with abnormal polarity where the diagnosis is usually retrospective. There is a focal circular ring of constriction in the inner muscle fibres at the upper and lower segment junction. It is not felt on abdominal examination and does not move upwards, unlike the pathological ring of obstructed labour. It is recognised while doing a caesarean section for failed descent in the second stage of labour or when forceps failed to deliver the fetus. During caesarean, the focal spasm restricts the delivery of the fetus, and either one must cut through the ring or deepen the anaesthesia to relax the spasmodic constriction to deliver the fetus.

The other clinical situation is after vaginal delivery of the foetus when the placenta gets retained. While performing manual removal under anaesthesia, one realises the hourglass constriction at the junction of the upper and the lower segment as the cause for the problem. Deepening the anaesthesia relieves the spasm and permits the surgeons hand to the upper segment to complete the procedure. Premature rupture of membranes, premature instrumentation, and overzealous use of oxytocin could trigger this condition. This condition usually does not exhaust the woman or compromise the fetus.

NORMAL POLARITY

UTERINE INERTIA

This can be primary or secondary. The uterine contractions are not strong enough to bring about cervical change. *Primary inertia* can happen in elderly, obese women, overdistension due to polyhydramnios, or multiple gestations. This can result in a prolonged latent phase.

Secondary inertia is a condition when after achieving the active phase of labour with good uterine contractions, the uterine contractions start reducing in intensity, frequency, and duration. It is more often seen in a primigravida. This is a protective mechanism against obstructed labour and ruptured uterus. Cephalo-pelvic disproportion, contracted pelvis, malpresentation and position, big baby, dehydration, maternal anxiety, and fear can cause this condition. A caesarean section might be necessary to deliver such a woman. Contracted pelvis and disproportion pelvis should be ruled out before considering augmenting with oxytocin. Otherwise, there can be disastrous consequences like obstructed labour, ruptured uterus, and arrest in the second stage.

Uterine tachysystole: The uterine contraction of more than 5 in 10 minutes is called tachysystole. It may or may not be accompanied by abnormalities of the fetal heart. Any contraction lasting more than 60 seconds is referred to as hypercontraction. Any excess uterine contractility accompanied by fetal heart rate abnormality was earlier referred to as hyperstimulation. Excessive use of oxytocics and not maintaining adequate gap between the cervical ripening agents such as prostaglandin E2 and the inducing agents such as oxytocin or prostaglandin E1 can cause tachysystole. Sometimes chorioamnionitis can also cause tachysystole.

Hyperstimulation needs to be corrected by intrauterine resuscitation. Intrauterine resuscitation includes changing the position to left lateral, intravenous infusion of crystalloid fluid and administration of oxygen by intranasal catheter or face mask. If the contractions do not reduce in duration and frequency, tocolytic agents like 0.25 mg terbutaline should be administered subcutaneously. With these measures, the fetal heart abnormality usually gets corrected.

Precipitate Labour

When the labour completes in less than 3 hours after the commencement of contractions, it is called precipitate labour. The strongest risk factor is a history of precipitate labour. It is more likely in multiparous women.

Abruptio placenta, meconium-stained liquor, cocaine abuse, and iatrogenic hyperstimulation with oxytocic can also result in precipitate labour. In a primipara teenage, hypertension, preterm labour, and low birth weight were found to be associated with precipitate labour.[5] The complications of preterm labour include trauma to the reproductive tract in the form of tears of the cervix, vaginal laceration, and postpartum haemorrhage due to atony as well as trauma. Precipitate labour can predispose to life-threatening complication of amniotic fluid embolism.

There is a risk of fetal trauma due to a fall if the delivery is unattended.

Cervical Dystocia

When the external os fails to dilate despite good uterine contractions, it is called cervical dystocia. It can be primary or secondary. It can occur when the cervix has undergone scarring due to previous surgery, infection, or trauma. Surgeries such as amputation or trachelorrhaphy, cauterisation, and trauma due to irradiation can predispose to fibrosis and dystocia. The healing process following illness and tears sustained at childbirth change the proportion of muscle and scar tissue in the cervix. Excess scar tissue prevents passive dilation of the cervix in labour. Women with uterovaginal prolapse in labour with the cervix lying outside can have a similar problem of cervical dystocia. Sacculation of the posterior wall of the uterus and the cervix, congenital absence of portio-vaginalis, cervical atresia, and cancer cervix are other causes of cervical dystocia.

In certain situations, even in the absence of any such previous influence, the cervix might fail to dilate despite good contractions. This condition is called primary cervical dystocia. The external os may fail to dilate secondary to cephalopelvic disproportion and poor alignment of the fetus to the axis of the cervix or inadequate pelvis (secondary dystocia). Therefore, in primary cervical dystocia, the fetal presenting part should be well engaged. The uterine contractions should be regular and good. The pelvis should also be normal and the cervix should be well effaced. At the level of the external os, a cicatrix or cartilaginous ring is often felt below which the cervix fails to dilate. The portion of the cervix above the ring area is often thinned out and stretched. In certain cases, it is a disorder of the function of the cervix (due to sympathetic overactivity or altered muscle proportion of the cervix), and the cicatrix may not be evident. Sometimes, the external os may be difficult to define and sometimes it may be pushed posteriorly to the sacrum. The treatment for dystocia of the cervix involves sedation and good hydration of the woman and reassessment after 2 hours. True dystocia invariable requires a caesarean section to deliver the fetus. The cervix may have to be dilated from above if it is completely stenosed. In certain cases of a prolapsed cervix where the upper part is thinned and dilated, Duhrssen's incision may be tried to cut the scarred thickened portion. In such situations, the incision should be placed around the 2 and 10 o'clock positions. Sometimes additional or only at 6 o'clock position is also likely to help. It has the risk of extension and formation of broad ligament hematoma and excessive bleeding.

OXYTOCIN

This is an octapeptide that is synthesised in the hypothalamus. It is then transported to the pituitary gland. The levels peak in labour and are released in pulses. Oxytocin increases the calcium levels in the myofibrils. The response and further release of oxytocin are influenced by the activation of the receptors on the myometrium. Positive feedback in labour enhances the recruitment of the oxytocin receptors on the myofibrils. After starting oxytocin infusion, the steady-state concentration in the plasma is reached by about 40–60 minutes, and the half-life is 1–6 minutes. The initiation labour with exogenous oxytocin can be through a low-dose or a high-dose regimen. The low-dose regimen starts at less than 2 mU/minute. The preterm uterus is less likely to respond to oxytocin and may require a higher dose to initiate labour. It is logical to understand that the induction of labour requires higher oxytocin doses compared to augmentation of contractions after spontaneous onset of uterine contractions.

Regimens of oxytocin: Induction at term in a nulliparous woman would require 2–6 mU/minute (high-dose regimen). Given the half-life of the oxytocin, it is important to understand that the oxytocin infusion rate should be escalated periodically. Dosing intervals followed vary from 15 to 40 minutes in various Institutions. It should be escalated at least every hour. Escalating every 30 minutes would yield an optimal response. Escalating earlier than that may cause hyperstimulation. The escalation can be either arithmetic with an increase by 1–2 mU every 30 minutes or exponential to the starting dose (for example, if starting is 1 mU/minute, then exponential increase means one increased to 2 followed by 4, 8, 16, 32, 64 mU/minute (doubling)). The problem with exponential increase is that it helps achieve the maximum dose faster but might prolong the time taken to achieve optimal uterine contractions and can cause hyperstimulation.

The arithmetic increase is preferred (1, 2, 4, 8, 12, 16, 20, 24, 28, 32 mU/minute). So the increase is by 4 mIU/min every 30 minutes. The product characteristics claim that 20 mIU is the licensed maximum dose. The clinical use with 32 is safe. In multigravida and women with a scarred uterus, we can down-regulate the dose of the oxytocin infusion after good regular contractions are established because positive feedback will increment the response. It is important to acknowledge that one must increase the dose every half hour till targeted contractions (3 to 5 contractions lasting 40 seconds in 10 minutes is achieved); otherwise, *tachyphylaxis* sets in. Tachyphylaxis is loss or weakening of response with escalating doses due to desensitisation of the receptors. Lower starting doses are preferred for augmentation. Short intervals of 15 minutes to increase the dose of oxytocin are associated with tachysystole. Longer than 40 minutes will result in tachyphylaxis.

One must understand that the biomolecular response of oxytocin is negatively influenced by dehydration/ketosis/electrolyte imbalance at the biomolecular level. So even though the women may not appear dehydrated, exhaustion of labour causing disturbed homeostasis at a cellular level can blunt the response to oxytocin. So many a time, the response to oxytocin can be improved by stopping the oxytocin drip and hydrating and nourishing the woman. Parenteral or epidural analgesia can also put the contractions and progress back to track by reducing the ketosis and electrolytes at a cellular level by relieving the pain.

O'Driscoll active management of labour or the Dublin protocol: This was described in 1984. The regimen included artificial rupture of membranes and initiating induction with a higher dose of 6 mIU/minute and escalated by 6 mIU/minute. Many studies have confirmed shorter induction to delivery interval and fewer failed inductions with this protocol.

The maximum dosage of oxytocin that can be used for induction of labour at term is 32 mIU/minute, and the contractions targeted are 200 Montevideo units. It is preferred to avoid more than 20 mIU/minute in the scarred uterus and multiparous women.

Doses higher than 20 mIU/minute are known to cause fluid retention and needs vigilance. When intravenous fluids have to be restricted, high-dose low-flow rate or infusion pumps can be used to administer oxytocin.

TIMELINE DEFINITIONS FOR ABNORMAL LABOUR

For consistency of identification of the problem and its management, it is important to understand the permitted upper time limits for defining problems of labour.

It is expected that cervical dilation must proceed at least 1 cm/hour after reaching the active phase of labour. The active stage is taken as at least 4 cm dilation. The definition has been changing. The Consortium of labour[6] has recommended that 6 cm dilation should be achieved before non-progress of labour is assigned as a reason for caesarean section. The reason being that the labour proceeds consistently above 1 cm/hour only after 6 cm and is likely to be slower than 1 cm/hour from 4 to 6 cm (Zhangs guidelines[7,8]). The WHO has recently recommended 5 cm dilation for defining active phase of labour.[9]

Prolonged latent phase: The highest cut-off for a prolonged latent phase of labour is taken as 20 hours in a nulliparous woman and 14 hours in a multiparous woman.

The active phase of labour: Labour should proceed at 1 cm/hour in nulliparous and anywhere from 1.2 to 1.5 cm/hour in a multiparous woman. The timelines depend on the definition taken for the onset of the active phase of labour. An active phase lasting longer than 12 hours in a nulliparous woman and longer than 6 hours in a multiparous woman is taken as abnormal and requires intervention.

Protracted dilation: As already mentioned, the expected rate of dilation after achieving the active phase of labour in a nulliparous woman is 1 to 1.2 cm/hour, and in a multigravida, it is about 1.5 cm/hour. Dilation slower than 0.5 cm/hour in a nullipara and slower than 0.8 cm/hour in a multiparous woman is taken as the cut-off for abnormality. If the deceleration phase was longer than 3 hour it was considered as prolonged. It was viewed as the arrest of dilation if there is no change in cervical dilation for 2 hours despite good contractions, but the definitions have changed: no change in cervix even after 4–6 hours of good contractions after the active phase is defined as *arrest of dilation*. In the recent WHO labour guide,[9] the definition of protracted dilation or arrested dilation has been revised to a duration longer than 6 hours at 5 cm dilation, 5 hours at 6 cm, 3 hours at 7 cm, 2.5 hours at 8 cm, and 2 hours or longer at 9 cm dilation.

Disorders of descent of the head: Ideally, descent proceeds at 1 cm/hour after the active phase of labour. However, the rate varies based on parity and the starting station. In a nulliparous woman, the head is usually at a lower station when the labour starts. If the head was already at 0 or −1 cm station, then most of the descent is likely to occur in the transition and second stages of labour. Earlier, no descent of head for 1 hour in a nulliparous woman and 2 hours in a multiparous woman was considered as the **arrest of descent**. And if there is no descent in the second stage, it was defined as **failed descent**. Recently the Consortium of labour[8] has redefined the failed descent. If after 3 hours of active pushing in a nulliparous and 2 hours of active pushing in a multiparous woman in the second stage, there is no descent and delivery is not completed, it is considered an arrest.

Such a situation needs reassessment for features of cephalopelvic disproportion and deflexion. Sometimes cord around the neck could be the reason for deflexion, and invariably, the fetus manifests distress with the cord loop getting tightened and dictates delivery by caesarean section. The arrest of descent in the second stage of labour warrants intervention by caesarean section if the station is above +1.

MANAGEMENT GOALS OF ABNORMAL LABOUR

Abnormal labour can be due to problem in the three "P"s: the passage, the passenger, and the power.

A pelvis that was thought to be normal might become inadequate for a slightly bigger baby or a fetus in occipitoposterior position. Deflexed head and compound presentation can also result in abnormal labour.

The uterine contractions impart the power to complete the fetal journey and help overcome problems due to malposition and borderline disproportion.

Any inertia or incoordinate action of the uterus after achieving the active stage of labour warrants thorough assessment of the other two "P"s. If the pelvis appears adequate and the fetus appears to be doing fine, and if features of disproportion have been ruled out, then correction of other subtle factors listed below is likely to correct the progress.

a. **Pain relief**: A suitable sedation or analgesia relieves pain and allays anxiety and is likely to correct the uterine contractions.

b. **Correction of dehydration**: Even though the woman may not appear dehydrated, there may be only mild tachycardia; there is likely to be dehydration at the cellular level. Quite often, we underestimate the fluid requirement, notwithstanding that she might have been in the labour room for long and might have been vomiting. Ensuring intravenous hydration with ringer lactate or normal saline helps to overcome this and helps to revert labour to normal.

c. **Nutrition**: Once again, this aspect is quite often ignored in the busy labour room, especially when the woman is undergoing induction of labour starting from an unfavourable cervix or has had a long latent phase and not eaten well. Ensuring good nutrition through oral fluids or a semiliquid diet is necessary. Allowing the woman to have some food sometimes even after achieving the active phase of labour may be worthwhile in a few selected group of women. A few women at higher risk of likely intrapartum caesarean might have been advised to remain nil oral. Those kept nil per oral should be kept well-nourished with intravenous dextrose to ensure adequate hydration and nourishment.

d. **Emotional support**: "A tense mind is a tense cervix" is a well-known adage. Taking the woman into confidence by counselling them about their condition, discussing their delivery plan, and periodically appraising the woman and the companion goes a long way in gaining their confidence and encourages them during labour. The process of counselling should start in the antenatal period itself. In the last few visits at term, antenatal visits should be spent explaining the benefits of vaginal delivery and clarifying their doubts and allaying any anxiety. I have experienced that woman who has a strong urge to deliver vaginally definitely succeed.

I would like to narrate a case: A second gravida with a previous spontaneous vaginal delivery was admitted with breech presentation at 39 weeks and 2 days of gestation. An external cephalic version had failed. All factors favoured a vaginal delivery, and she was very motivated for a vaginal delivery. We had counselled her that we will not induce her, but if she does not go into spontaneous labour by 41 weeks, we will do a caesarean section. She went into labour and delivered the night before she was planned for elective caesarean section.

Recognising this need for internal motivation in a woman to deliver vaginally, I have started spending more time with the woman in the last few antenatal visits talking to them about normal delivery and its advantages. Sometimes I suggest they do positive imagery and I also do positive visualisation that they are normally delivering when they are in labour.

e. **Artificial rupture of membranes (ARM)**: This should be usually performed after the woman enters the active phase. It may be necessary for a few women before 4 cm dilation. Woman undergoing induction of labour, including those with previous caesarean section benefit with an early ARM when performed with the onset of regular uterine contractions and even with a 2–3 cm dilation. It not only enhances labour but also reveals the colour of liquor which may be necessary when the risk of meconium or abruption is high. O'Driscoll had introduced the concept of active management of labour way back in the 70s. A lot of obstetricians do not like to perform ARM even after achieving the active phase of labour. In my view, ARM is a particularly important armamentarium for labour management. Done in the right woman at the right time works wonders. The softness and effacement in a nulliparous woman and the dilation of 2–3 cm in the presence of regular uterine contractions usually favour the response to ARM. It should be used with prudence and liberally in women with severe preeclampsia or eclampsia and women with previous caesarean sections undergoing labour induction. I prefer to do ARM for all woman in the active phase of labour. It should not be done to prevent delayed labour or in the latent phase if there is no indication to worry or accelerate labour.

Controlled ARM may be necessary in certain cases of brim trial and polyhydramnios. ARM helps fix the head in brim trials and helps to observe the signs of abnormal labour. It should be performed preferably in the active phase of labour in the brim trial.

ARM in polyhydramnios relieves the overdistension and corrects incoordinate uterine activity due to overdistension. Cord prolapse and abruption are distinct complications. It can be prevented in polyhydramnios by doing controlled ARM with the prick of a long 26 gauze needle shielded with a cannula (like the spinal needle or intravenous cannula needle) held in the left hand and guided by the finger of the right hand. The pricked point should be quickly covered with the gloved sterile finger of the right hand, and the fluid should be allowed to escape slowly. Sometimes it may take 10–20 minutes to allow the slow escape of liquor. This procedure should never be hurried up. Sudden decompression of the uterus can cause abruption. We need to allow time for the presenting part to fix to prevent cord prolapse..

f. **Oxytocin augmentation**: Augmentation with oxytocin might be necessary if the contractions are not optimal. In woman already undergoing augmentation or induction of labour, it is particularly important to understand tachyphylaxis (as explained in the previous section). If the oxytocin drip rate is not escalated every 20–30 minutes till effective contractions are reached, then the effect of an ongoing dose of oxytocin gets attenuated over time, and the contractions slowly become less intense. In such a situation, it is a good idea to restart oxytocin from a lower dose and escalate every half an hour till the optimum response is achieved. Sometimes it is a good idea to give a short break for hydration and nutrition before restarting the oxytocin drip.

g. **Reassess the case**: Thus, the management strategy for abnormal labour depends on reviewing the case for understanding the reason behind the abnormal progress. One must assess the fetal position, features of cephalopelvic disproportion, the reason for erratic uterine activity, and carefully reassess the pelvis for its type and tendency at all three levels. The uterus's good and fruitful power can be ensured by keeping the woman in a good state of hydration, nutrition, and pain relief to ensure good physical, mental, metabolic, and emotional stamina.

Sometimes even with the best of the above efforts, including ARM, the labour does not progress, and the uterine contractions may remain incoordinate or inadequate. I just wonder if this is a subtle alert from nature and forewarning from the uterus against vaginal delivery. Quite often, to our surprise, the fetus turns out to be much heavier than suspected. If eventually full dilation was achieved, the delivery ends up as a complicated instrumental delivery or many loops of tight cord around the neck that was not suspected antenatally.

COMPLICATIONS OF ABNORMAL LABOUR: ABNORMAL LABOUR CAN RESULT IN CERTAIN COMPLICATIONS ENUMERATED BELOW

a. Maternal exhaustion
b. Fetal distress, hypoxia, acidosis
c. Chorioamnionitis
d. Arrest in the second stage of labour
e. Failed instrumental delivery
f. Difficult caesarean section with uterine incision extension
g. PPH and maternal sepsis
h. Birth asphyxia (severe hypoxic-ischaemic encephalopathy can result in long-term neurological sequel)
i. Early-onset neonatal sepsis
j. Meconium aspiration syndrome
k. Increased risk of stillbirth and neonatal death

Thus, being proactive in recognising that labour has become abnormal, reassessing the case to discover the reason behind the abnormality, and instituting remedial measures and continued surveillance of labour is needed to manage abnormal labour.

REFERENCES

1. Tilden EI, Phillippi JC, Ahlberg M, et al. Describing latent phase duration and associated characteristics among 1281 low-risk women in spontaneous labor. *Birth.* 2019;46(4):592–601. doi:10.1111/birt.12428.
2. Rosenbloom JI, Woolfolk CL, Wan L, et al. The transition from latent to active labor and adverse obstetrical outcomes. *Am J Obstet Gynecol.* 2019;221(5):487.e1–487.e8. doi:10.1016/j.ajog.2019.05.041.
3. Ängeby K, Wilde-Larsson B, Hildingsson I, Sandin-Bojö AK. Prevalence of prolonged latent phase and labor outcomes: Review of birth records in a Swedish population. *J Midwifery Women's Health.* 2018;63(1):33–44. doi:10.1111/jmwh.12704.
4. Roth C, Dent SA, Parfitt SE, Hering SL, Bay RC. Randomized controlled trial of use of the peanut ball during labor. *MCN Am J Matern Child Nurs.* 2016;41(3):140–146.
5. Suzuki S. Clinical significance of precipitous labor. *J Clin Med Res.* 2015 Mar;7(3):150–153. doi: 10.14740/jocmr2058w. Epub 2014 Dec 29. PMID: 25584099; PMCID: PMC4285060.
6. Safe Pevention of Primary Caesarean Delivery. Obstetric Care Consensus No.1, American College of Obstetrics and Gynecologists. *Obstete Gynecol.* 2014;123: 693–711.
7. Bernitz S, Dalbye R, Zhang J, et al. The frequency of intrapartum caesarean section use with the WHO partograph versus Zhang's guideline in the Labour Progression Study (LaPS): A multicentre, cluster-randomised controlled trial. *Lancet.* 2019;393(10169):340–348. doi:10.1016/S0140-6736(18)31991-3
8. Zhang J Troendle J Mikolajczyk R Sundaram R Beaver J Fraser W. The natural history of the normal first stage of labor. *Obstet Gynecol.* 2010;115: 705–710.
9. WHO. *WHO Labour Care Guide: User's Manual. Geneva: World Health Organization*; 2020. Licence: CC BY-NC-SA 3.0 IGO. WHO. Accessed on December 14 2020.

12 Cephalopelvic Disproportion and Contracted Pelvis

Gowri Dorairajan
Jawaharlal Institute of Postgraduate Medical
Education and Research (JIPMER)

Dimensional or mechanical disparity between the fetus and the pelvis is called cephalopelvic disproportion (CPD). The fetus is considered the best pelvimeter. Normal labour, unfortunately, is a retrospective diagnosis. An engaged head rules out contraction at the level of the inlet. An unengaged head in a primigravida is always a cause of anxiety to the care provider and the woman alike. It is important to acknowledge that the head usually engages before the onset of labour in a primigravida. However, in the absence of a low-lying placenta, deflexed head, cord around the neck, and lower segment fibroids, a free-floating head in a primigravida should raise suspicion of CPD that is likely to manifest in labour.

Labour is the true test for disproportion. The ability to predict with reasonable surety if labour will complete itself uneventfully is incredibly challenging. There are various clinical as well as objective imaging techniques for predicting successful vaginal delivery. Most of the clinical methods are tests to screen in for trial labour. Passing the clinical screening does not guarantee successful vaginal delivery. It only gives a fair idea that it is likely to succeed. Continued vigilance is necessary to detect manifest features of disproportion making the labour abnormal. Let us learn the clinical methods for the fit of the head as a screening for allowing trial of labour

CLINICAL IDENTIFICATION TESTS

The clinical tests are not confirmatory. Labour is the best pelvimeter. Clinical methods help us triaging and increasing our vigil on the borderline cases during labour to look for various signs of CPD carefully.

These clinical methods for assessment of CPD can be abdominal only or bimanual. The methods are as below:

    a. Chasar Moir
    b. **Muller-Kerr** method
    c. Pinard's method
    d. Donald's method
    e. Purandare's method

These are detailed below.

Chassar Moir method (Figure 12.1): This is an external method. It is carried out by standing on the woman's right side, the woman being in a dorsal position. The head is held by the thumb and the palm of the left hand. The index and middle finger of the right hand rest horizontally over the upper border of the pubis symphysis. With gentle downward pressure by the left hand, if the head can be made to enter the pelvis under the pubic symphysis, it rules out major disproportion. However, if the head tends to touch or override the fingers on the pubic symphysis on downward push, then features of CPD should be watched out for during labour.

DOI: 10.1201/9781003034360-12

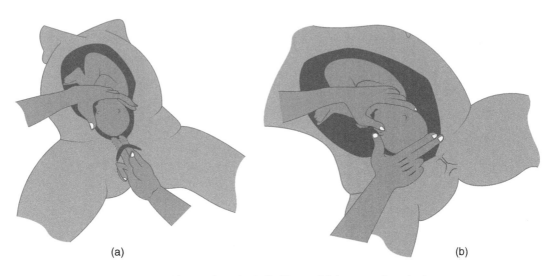

(a)   (b)

FIGURE 12.1   (a) Muller-Kerr bimanual method. (b) Chassar Moir external method.

Muller–Kerr method (Figure 12.1): This is a bimanual method carried out with the woman in a dorsal position. The gloved index and the middle finger of the right hand of the obstetrician are introduced in the vagina under aseptic precautions. The thumb is placed over the pubic symphysis. So, this method can be undertaken before withdrawing fingers from the vagina during digital examination for pelvic assessment and ripening score assessment.

The head which is above the brim is held externally by the left hand between the thumb and the fingers. Gentle downward pressure on the head is given by the left hand. If the vaginal fingers feel the head to negotiate to enter the brim, then serious disproportion is unlikely. However, if head flushes, then mild, and if it overrides the pubic symphysis, then serious disproportion is likely and requires vigilance in labour.

Pinard's method: This is an external method carried out in a semi-sitting position. The idea is to ensure that the fetal axis is perpendicular to the inlet of the brim while pushing the head downwards gently as one tests for the fit of the head.

Donald's method: This is also an external method with the woman in a dorsal position. Here the knees are slightly flexed, and a pillow is kept below the shoulders. The fingers of both hands hold the sinciput and occiput on either side. Both the index fingers rest on the upper limit of the pubic symphysis. The thumbs are over the parietal eminence of the head. Pushing the head from above with the hands while facing the legs of the woman will give an idea of the fit of the head to the inlet of the pelvis.

Purandare's method: Purandare described the external method as mentioned under the Chassar Moir methods but in an extended lithotomy position.

The inference of all the above methods is similar. The above describe methods are screening method and help us suspect minor or likely serious disproportion and alert us for the need for vigilance in labour. In women with serious disproportion, labour should be avoided, especially if the baby is big and the internal pelvimetry reveals a contracted pelvis.

EXTERNAL PELVIMETRY

The landmarks are the highest point on the iliac crest, the anterior superior iliac spines, the posterior superior iliac spines, the ischial tuberosity, upper border of the pubic symphysis, the fifth lumbar spinous process, and the beginning of the intergluteal fold (representing the tip of the sacrum). The following clinical pelvimetry has been described.

Inter-anterior superior iliac spine distance (Interspinous diameter) less than 25 cm and/or
Inter-crestal diameter (between the two farthest points on the Iliac crest) less than 28 cm
External conjugate (Baudeloque's diameter): The distance between the upper border of the
  pubic symphysis and the first sacral segment less than 20 cm should raise a suspicion of
  the pelvic capacity.
The base of the Trillats triangle and the transverse diameter of the Michaels rhomboid area
  have been measured.

These diameters can be measured with a steel calliper called an external pelvimeter (example, the
Collins pelvimeter). External pelvimetry is clinically obsolete and cumbersome.

Various measurements are taken in different positions like the kneel up position, all four and the
kneel squat position. In a study[1], the authors observed that the diameters are increased in all four
and the kneel squat position. These are also the generally preferred positions by the woman. The
dorsal position with the hips hyper-flexed serves similarly to increase the diameters.

Dynamic external pelvimetry is cumbersome and not routinely followed in modern obstetrics.

X-RAY PELVIMETRY

This involves taking at least two X-ray films: one anteroposterior in the supine position and another
lateral view in the standing position.

The dimensions described are the maximum transverse, median transverse, and promontory to
the posterior surface of the symphysis pubis distance. The Magnin index is the sum of the last two.
Magnin index of more than 23 cm was found to have a good prognosis for vaginal delivery. 90.74%
concordance was found in women classified as unfavourable prognosis on X-ray pelvimetry based on
the various diameters calculated[2]. In a study, X-ray was taken postpartum among women recruited
antenatally. The authors[3] observed that at the plane of ischial spines, the anteroposterior diameter
<9.5 cm (area under ROC of 0.88) and the circumference at this plane <29.8 cm (area under ROC of
0.85) predicted caesarean section more accurately than the transverse diameter less than 9 cm at the
same plane (area under ROC of 0.65). They measured the anteroposterior diameter from the third
sacral vertebra.

The recently published Cochrane review[4] analysed the studies comparing X-ray pelvimetry with
no pelvimetry or clinical pelvimetry. The authors concluded against the use of X-ray pelvimetry to
decide the mode of delivery in women with cephalic presentation.

ROLE OF CT SCAN AND MRI

MRI is taken in three planes to measure the obstetric conjugate, interspinous distance, sagittal diameter from the tip of the sacrum to the lower aspect of the pubic symphysis, the inter-tuberosity distance,
and the widest transverse diameter at the inlet. In a study[5], the obstetric conjugate, interspinous, widest
transverse at the inlet, and the anteroposterior of the outlet were significantly lesser in those who had a
caesarean delivery. The anteroposterior outlet diameter has been consistently reported to be lesser with
MRI than with X-ray, probably due to the positioning. Sagittal midpelvic diameter of 12.7 + 0.6 cm on
abdominal CT scan was found to have 85% sensitivity and specificity for predicting CPD[6].

Low-dose stereo radiographic imaging: This was found to be as accurate and with 13 times
lower radiation dose to the fetus and three times lower exposure to the pregnant woman.[7]

CONTRACTED PELVIS

Any dimension of the pelvis is so narrow that normal delivery is not possible, then it is called a
contracted pelvis. Anatomically, it is a reduction in one or the other diameter by more than 1 cm
below the normal.

The contracted pelvis can occur at any or all the three levels, viz. the inlet, the plane of least pelvic dimensions (also called as mid pelvic contraction), and the anatomical outlet. Let us learn more about this at the various levels in detail.

Objective Definition for Contracted Pelvis

Inlet Contraction

The transverse diameter compensates for any narrowing of the anteroposterior diameter at the inlet. The area of the plane of the inlet (transverse × anteroposterior diameter) should be ideally more than 120 cm^2 (Mengerts index). When the surface area at the plane of the inlet is less than 95 square cm, it is taken as a contracted pelvis. It is not easy to clinically measure the transverse diameter unless external pelvimetry is done to note the distance between the anterior superior iliac spines. The Magnin index (sum of AP and transverse diameter at inlet) should be more than 23 cm on X-ray. The fetopelvic index, which takes on imaging, compares the fetal head and abdominal circumference with the maternal inlet and outlet measurement. From a single clinical dimension point of view, if diagonal conjugate that is measured at the time of pelvic assessment is found to be less than 11.5 cm (which means the obstetric conjugate is less than 10 cm), it is defined as contracted brim. Serious dystocia occurs if the obstetric conjugate is less than 9 cm or the surface area of the inlet is less than 90 cm^2.

Midpelvic Contraction

This refers to contraction at the plane of least pelvic dimension. If the sum of the interischial spine diameter and the posterior sagittal diameter is less than 13.5 cm, it is considered inadequate and qualifies as mid pelvic contraction. An interischial spine diameter of less than 10 cm is considered borderline, and less than 9 cm also signifies mid pelvic contraction. Normally, this diameter exceeds 15.5 cm. The subpubic angle can compensate for posterior sagittal diameter at the plane of least pelvic dimensions. The assessment must be thorough with attention to the interischial spine diameter and the posterior sagittal diameter (distance between the sacrococcygeal joint and a line drawn between the two ischial spines), especially so in occipital-posterior positions.

Outlet Contraction

Isolated contraction at the anatomical outlet alone is exceedingly rare. The anatomical outlet is said to be contracted when the transverse diameter of the outlet is less than 8 cm. The same is reflected by a narrow pubic arch (angle less than 85°).

The four parent type of pelvis has been already discussed in Chapter 1. There could be combinations of one parent type at the upper part with a tendency to another type in the lower part of the pelvis.

The android is a contracted pelvis and likely to result in severe dystocia and arrest in the mid pelvis. The anthropoid pelvis is more likely to be associated with malposition. Face to pubes delivery is a more likely fate in the anthropoid pelvis.

CAUSES FOR CONTRACTED PELVIS

Contracted pelvis can occur due to
Abnormalities of the spine or diseases of the pelvic bone and joints.

These can happen due to:

- Nutritional deficiency.
- Congenital abnormalities.
- Acquired diseases like tuberculosis.
- Trauma to the concerning bones.

I will discuss a few of these in detail.

ABNORMALITIES OF THE SPINE

Spine has an important function of weight-bearing in adults. The weight is transmitted to the pelvis from the spine and to both femur through the pelvis. The spinal abnormalities can affect the curvature, changing the dynamics of the sacral promontory and the sacrum. Deformities in the lumbosacral spine are more likely to affect the pelvis.

Kyphosis: This means abnormal outward curvature of the spine. It pulls the sacral promontory backwards and outwards and tilts the coccyx forwards.

The anteroposterior diameter of the inlet increases but that of the anatomical outlet decreases. The plane of the inlet becomes more horizontal. As pregnancy advances to term, there can be malalignment of the fetal axis to the inlet of the pelvis. This can get worse due to a pendulous abdomen resulting from vertebral column deformity. The sacrum often is flat and straight. The transverse diameter is slightly narrow at the inlet, and the trend continues till the outlet. So, while the brim is anteroposterior oval, the outlet may be contracted. Thus, isolated outlet contraction can occur in lumbar spine kyphosis and requires careful assessment of this level to prevent surprise arrest in the second stage of labour.

Suppose the kyphosis is higher up in the thoracic spine (tubercular gibbus is a common cause in India), In that case, compensatory lordosis may develop in the lumbar spine, making the inlet more vertical than usual and with an increased anteroposterior diameter.

One also needs to keep in mind that the abnormalities of the thoracic spine are likely to be associated with compromised respiratory and cardiac reserve and function.

Scoliosis: Lateral curvature of the spine is of obstetric significance only when severe and in the lumbar spine. It can bring about deflection of the sacral promontory to one side and make the brim irregular. In association with rickets, it may assume serious obstetric significance at the level of the brim of the pelvis.

Spondylolisthesis: A condition where the last lumbar vertebra (L5) slips down in front of the sacral S1 vertebra. This results in a false promontory and reduces the anteroposterior diameter at the brim of the pelvis. Depending on the degree of affection, there may be a serious compromise of the obstetric conjugate.

ABNORMALITIES OF THE PELVIS AND THE JOINTS

Nutritional Disorders: Rickets and osteomalacia are the most typical disorders affecting the mineralisation of the bones. This results in soft bones, which tend to deform easily due to pressures of weight-bearing.

Rachitic pelvis: Vitamin D deficiency is an important problem in childhood days, especially in developing countries. The distortion or changes in the pelvis depend on the age at which the child was affected because the weight-bearing part of the body is different at different ages. A child from 10 months to 2 years is more often sitting, whereas children more than 2 years is more likely to be standing and walking through the day.

In a more often sitting child, the weight is transmitted through the spine to the pelvis and the ischial tuberosity. If the child is affected with rickets in such an age group, the weight-bearing in sitting position affects the soft sacrum. The sacral promontory gets pushed downwards and forwards and the coccyx backwards. The sacrospinous ligament may try to restrain the pushing back of the sacral tip and may cause a sharp bending at the sacrococcygeal joint. It may not be so obvious in a child who is more often lying down. The posterior iliac spines are dragged closer due to the stronger posterior sacroiliac ligaments. Therefore, the obstetric diagonal significantly decreases. The iliac bones are flared out, thereby increasing the inter-anterior superior iliac spine distance. This results in the increased transverse diameter of the inlet of the pelvis. The distance between the ischial spines also increases. So, a typical rachitic pelvis in a woman who was affected with rickets below 2 years of age would result in serious shortening of the anteroposterior diameter of the brim and increased transverse diameter of the brim resulting in a reniform shape of the inlet of the pelvis.

When the coccyx is pushed backwards, then the anteroposterior diameter is increased at the outlet. The flaring outwards of the iliac and ischial bone increases the transverse diameter from the inlet down to the outlet. So, the problem in such a pelvis is only at the inlet, and if the fetus negotiates the brim, then the rest of the journey of the fetus becomes easy because of a progressively spacious pelvis towards the mid and outlet.

In an elder child or adolescent more often standing or walking through the day, the weight-bearing occurs differently. The weight is borne by the spine and transmitted to the pelvis. As the bones are deformable, the sacral promontory juts forwards and reduces the obstetric conjugate. The pelvis transmits the weight to the femur through the hip joint. The sidewall of the pelvis at the femoral-pelvic joint succumbs to the forces, and the inward push by the acetabulum compromises the mid pelvis at the level of the plane of least pelvic dimensions. The sidewalls get pushed inside, causing beaking and narrowing anteriorly. The attachment of the rectus abdominis muscle to the pubic symphysis also accentuates the beaking anteriorly. The result is a triangular-shaped brim and a trifoliate or clove-shaped or triradiate pelvis. The side walls are converging, and the subpubic arch is narrow. This condition affecting women in adulthood is called *osteomalacia*. In addition to the above findings, her stature and height reduce due to the sinking of the trunk. This may be the reason for serious dystocia in a multigravida who has had previous uneventful vaginal deliveries. A high index of suspicion is necessary for multipara with poor nutrition and swinging gait.

The condition may go unsuspected due to previous normal delivery and may go unrecognised. If the dystocia is unrecognised, it may go on to rupture the uterus. A thorough pelvis assessment before the onset of labour in such women can prevent obstetric maladies.

The affection of an adolescent with overeating and an unbalanced diet can result in obesity associated with vitamin deficiency. The above deformation in the pelvis can get exaggerated due to excess weight.

Diseases affecting the bones and joints: Various problems like traumatic fractures and tuberculosis of the hip joint can affect the pelvis. Tuberculous arthritis of the sacroiliac joint can distort the ala of the sacrum and distort the brim of the pelvis. Tuberculosis of the femoral-pelvis joint can affect weight-bearing. It can distort the plane of least pelvis dimensions due to asymmetric weight-bearing. Fracture of the pelvis with resulting malunion or new bone formation during the healing process can cause asymmetry and alter the inner contour of the mid pelvis. The degree and level of distortion are dependent on the severity and the site of the affected bone or joint.

Polio: The residual muscle paralysis in childhood days can affect the pelvis. The weak muscles often result in abduction flexion and external rotation of the hip joint. This can cause pelvic obliquity and a lumbar lordosis to compensate.

Shortening of the limbs due to residual paralysis will alter the weight-bearing and cause asymmetry at the level of the plane of least pelvic dimensions.

CONGENITAL DEFORMITIES

Congenital absence of the ala of the sacrum will reduce the transverse diameter of the brim of the pelvis. If it affects only one ala (Naegle's Pelvis), there will be asymmetric contraction, and if it affects both the alae, then there will be a serious compromise of the transverse diameter of the inlet of the pelvis.

Assimilation pelvis: There may be a genetic variation in the formation of the sacrum. Six instead of five vertebrae may form the sacrum. This deepens the sacrum, and hence the pelvis increases the anteroposterior diameter of the pelvic brim and makes it high inclined.

If only four vertebrae constitute the sacrum, then the inclination of the brim is reduced, and the pelvis becomes shallow.

These subtle findings may be missed in inexperienced hands. In women with tardy progress or arrested progress after achieving the active phase of labour, one needs to carefully reassess for any of these missed findings during the reassessment.

TRIAL OF LABOUR

Trial of labour is nothing but allowing labour in a woman with a borderline pelvis with the hope of achieving a normal vaginal delivery. The trial of labour should be properly supervised. In a primigravida, a trial of labour is worth the effort as it can avert a scheduled caesarean section and give her a chance of vaginal delivery.

Goal: The goal is to achieve vaginal delivery without adversely affecting maternal and fetal well-being and should not increase maternal or perinatal morbidity or mortality.

Contraindications of a trial of labour:

1. **Contracted pelvis**: If the pelvis is contracted based on the objective definitions above, then there should be no trial of labour.
2. There is no role of a trial of labour in a woman with **mid pelvic or outlet contraction** for the simple reason the contraction at these levels manifests as dystocia or arrest late in labour and the second stage of labour. So, a failed trial would compromise fetal health due to prolonged labour and its associated asphyxia and sepsis and make caesarean delivery necessary in the second stage, which is associated with greatly increased morbidity to the woman.
3. There is no role of trial labour in women with **previous caesarean section**. We are not only trying the pelvis but also the scar. Prolonged labour, oxytocin infusion, failed trial, etc. can increase the risk of scar rupture.
4. For reasons quite understandable, there is no role of trial labour in women with **severe preeclampsia and diabetes with macrosomia**.
5. **Previous bad obstetric outcome**: Women with previous prolonged labour and difficult instrumental delivery and who have delivered stillborn or asphyxiated babies due to prolonged labour should not be subjected to trial of labour.
6. Women with **breech presentation** should not be subjected to trial as there is not enough time for the head to mould and overcome a borderline pelvis.
7. It may not be prudent to try labour if the pelvis is borderline in **elderly women** who **conceived after many attempts through artificial reproductive techniques**, those who have recurrent pregnancy losses, or bad obstetric history.

Therefore, a trial of labour is generally advocated in women with borderline contraction of the inlet (brim) of the pelvis. The flat pelvis and rachitic pelvis have a good chance of delivering if the brim is negotiated as the inlet is the level of problem and the rest of the pelvis is spacious. Thus, there is a scope of trial labour only for suspected or borderline brim contraction.

MANAGEMENT OF TRIAL LABOUR

The goal of trial labour is to ensure delivery without increasing maternal or perinatal morbidity or mortality.

Counselling the woman and her partner about the plan, the likelihood of success, and the need for emergency caesarean in case of a failed trial are important to gain cooperation and allay anxiety. An effective enema to empty the rectum before the induction of labour or at the onset of labour would help reduce contamination and help achieve the best possible available diameters in the pelvis.

The trial should be undertaken *in a setup* that has the facility for caesarean section round the clock, adequate staff, anaesthetist and blood bank, electronic fetal monitoring, and expertise to monitor the labour for signs of a failed trial. It may be prudent to refer the woman for trial to an appropriate centre instead of delivering by elective prelabour caesarean section in the absence of the required facilities.

As we embark on trial labour, it is vital to understand that the triad of hypoxia, infection, and meconium in liquor can cause serious adverse perinatal outcomes, especially when combined.

Thus, *preventing infection* is a necessary precaution. In this regard, multiple vaginal examinations by different people should be avoided. Scrupulous antiseptic precautions are mandated for every digital examination. An early artificial rupture of membranes may not be a good idea as it might limit the length of labour and concern for infection may prompt premature decision for termination by caesarean section even before active labour is established. Antibiotics should be administered after rupturing of membranes. Speculum examination in the last weeks of antenatal check-up can help in detecting asymptomatic infection and provide adequate time to treat the infection appropriately before labour is induced.

Monitoring of labour: The labour should be monitored diligently with conscious awareness of the time frame for the progress of labour. Spontaneous labour is a favourable sign as natural forces achieve the best synchronised contraction power of the uterus.

Instead of repeated digital examination, the abdominal method to determine the descent of the head by palpating for the fifths of the head above the pubic symphysis (Notelovitz technique) can give a fair idea about the station of the head. The digital examination needs to be performed every 2 or 4 hours only after regular moderate uterine contractions have been established. Every digital examination to assess labour progress must be preceded by a good abdominal examination to note down the frequency, intensity, duration, and regularity of uterine contraction, rule out incoordinate uterine activity, and note the tone and relaxation of the uterus between contractions. One should also note the fifths of the head palpable above the brim. The fetal heart rate pattern should be noted before, during, and after a contraction in case of intermittent auscultation.

Every digital examination should be performed with scrupulous antiseptic measures. One must consciously note down the findings such as position, degree of flexion, moulding (if yes, then the grade and score), presence of caput, colour and amount of liquor draining beside the dilation, effacement, and suppleness of the cervix.

Progressive dilatation after the active phase of labour is established, and the partograph remaining to the left of the alert line is a reassuring finding to continue the trial. The fetal heart should be monitored diligently with intermittent auscultation or electronic monitoring to ensure fetal well-being. Prolonged recurrent early deceleration is suggestive of excessive head compression and indicates CPD.

In a woman undergoing induction of labour, one must ensure a mature cervix with a good Bishop score. Cervical ripening agents should be used with caution. Mechanical dilators like Foley catheter should be properly inserted to prevent converting the cephalic presentation to oblique or transverse lie and prevent cord prolapse from occurring.

Four hours of good uterine contraction (200 Montevideo units) after the woman has achieved the active phase of labour is necessary to affect a progress/show feature of CPD.

Artificial rupture of membranes (ARM) is an important intervention. It not only augments labour but also helps in the detection of caput, moulding and of course, the presence of meconium. However, a controlled ARM should be performed after regular uterine contraction has been established and a cervix is at least 3 cm dilated. Preventing cord prolapse when the head is above the brim is an important principle guiding the procedure. Too early, an ARM may not be prudent as it may compromise the time available for the trial, increase the risk of infection, reduce the cushioning effect to the fetal cord, and pose a cord prolapse threat.

Augmentation of labour in a woman who spontaneously achieves the active phase of labour should be done with caution. The oxytocin administration should start with a low dose and carefully titrated to achieve the target contractions.

One should spend time monitoring the pattern of uterine contraction to diagnose incoordinate contractions or secondary inertia requiring progressively higher doses of oxytocin. Avoid injudicious use of oxytocin or prostaglandin to prevent incoordinate contraction as well as tachysystole.

Adequate hydration and nutrition must be maintained. One must remember that she may have to remain nil per oral with the possibility of a need for an emergency caesarean section. So intravenous hydration and nutrition must be ensured, and women should be encouraged to pass urine. Adequate urination reassures the hydration status and helps keep the urinary bladder empty, which helps in fetal descent through the borderline brim.

Analgesia: There is no contraindication to epidural analgesia during the trial of labour. It should be timed after the onset of good uterine contractions. Parental opioids should be liberally used where epidural analgesia is not feasible. Adequate analgesia reduces anxiety, fear, and exhaustion occurring due to pain. This helps gain her cooperation in the trial of labour.

Mode of delivery: The goal of a trial of labour is to ensure the safe delivery of the fetus without adversely increasing fetal and maternal morbidity.

One should not hesitate to terminate by caesarean section even at full dilation instead of giving in to the temptation to use difficult instrumental delivery. A careful assessment of the station is necessary. There should be no palpable pole. Misjudgement of the station due to a large pelvic caput is a common mistake and a cause for the failed instrument. Taking a second opinion may reduce this error. Operative vaginal delivery should be undertaken only when all the prerequisites are fulfilled. In the situation of onset of spontaneous labour and satisfactory progress, a spontaneous vaginal delivery can be anticipated.

The endpoint of a trial of labour:

Diligent monitoring and record of the abdominal examination, the strength and pattern of uterine contractions, and the internal examination details (as mentioned earlier) will help pick up early signs of abnormal labour. This will help decide on the termination of the trial favouring emergency caesarean section at the right time without increasing maternal morbidity and jeopardising fetal well-being.

Following are the endpoints of trial labour:

1. Even after 6 hours of good uterine contraction in the active phase of labour, if the progress of labour is arrested or protracted progress (cervical dilation or descent).
2. Even after 6–8 hours of good uterine contractions after ARM, the woman fails to achieve active labour.
3. Moulding more than or equal to 4/6 or 7/9.
4. Large pelvic caput.
5. Meconium-stained liquor recognised before the active phase of labour or in combination with the above abnormal findings.
6. *Secondary inertia of uterus*: So, when any women whose requirement of oxytocin keeps on increasing after reaching the active phase of labour, one needs to assess for any alerting findings carefully. A primigravida would develop secondary inertia as a protective phenomenon. This language of the uterus needs to be recognised and respected. Whipping the uterus with injudicious use of oxytocin might help achieve full dilation but may bring labour to a standstill in the second stage.
7. *Abnormal fetal heart rate pattern*: Recurrent prolonged or severe early deceleration signifies head compression due to significant disproportion. Any suspicious or pathological fetal heart rate pattern is of concern in trial labour and needs emergency caesarean delivery, especially if the intrauterine resuscitation is not effective in reversing the pattern. I attribute this indication to fetal intelligence that may be far more than that of the monitoring obstetrician. However, some fetuses do sense the likely trouble and manifest distress much before the other features of dystocia come up, making the decision for caesarean delivery extremely easy. In these cases, during caesarean section, one may not find any placental or cord-related factors attributable to the distress.

8. Signs of cervical lips becoming thicker and hanging loose in the active phase are early subtle disproportion and merit termination features.

9. Intrapartum pyrexia more than 38°C is of concern in women after rupturing membranes in the absence of prostaglandin E1 analogues. As mentioned earlier, intrapartum infection in combination with hypoxia due to prolonged labour can worsen the perinatal outcome.

Thus, with good vigilance of the fetal and maternal condition, early detection of abnormal labour, ensuring proper selection of case for an assisted vaginal birth, and willingness to terminate by trial forceps or caesarean section in the second stage can give fruitful result for woman undergoing a trial of labour.

REFERENCES

1. Siccardi M, Valle C, Di Matteo F, et al. A postural approach to the pelvic diameters of obstetrics: The dynamic external pelvimetry test. *Cureus* 2019;11(11):e6111. doi:10.7759/cureus.6111.

2. Adisso S, Atrevy N, Adisso EL, Mukanire, Perrin RX, Alihonou E. X-ray pelvimetry: Prognosis of delivery by cephalous-pelvic confrontation in Cotonou. *Int J Reprod Contracept Obstet Gynecol* 2017;6:3737–41.

3. Harper LM, Odibo AO, Stamilio DM, Macones GA. Radiographic measures of the mid pelvis to predict cesarean delivery. *Am J Obstet Gynecol* 2013;208(6):460.e1–6. doi: 10.1016/j.ajog.2013.02.050. Epub 2013 Mar 1. PMID: 23467050; PMCID: PMC3672361.

4. Pattinson RC, Cuthbert A, Vannevel V. Pelvimetry for fetal cephalic presentations at or near term for deciding on mode of delivery. *Cochrane Database of Syst Rev* 2017;3(3): CD000161. doi: 10.1002/14651858.CD000161.

5. Fakher D, Marouf T, Azab AO. Value of magnetic resonance imaging in predicting cephalopelvic disproportion in relation to obstetric outcome: a pilot study. *J Evidence-Based Women's Health J Soc.* 2012;2(1):14–7. doi: 10.1097/01.EBX.0000410711.19975.69.

6. Miriam SL, Thorsten RCJ, Sabine W, Konstantin N, Klaus F, Uwe H. Pelvimetry revisited: Analysing cephalopelvic disproportion. *Euro J Radiol.* 2010;74(3): E107–11. https://doi.org/10.1016/j.ejrad.2009.04.042.

7. S. Aubry, P. Padoin, Y. Petegnief, C. Vidal, D. Riethmuller, E. Delabrousse three-dimensional pelvimetry using low-dose stereoradiography replace low-dose CT pelvimetry? *Diagn Interv Imaging.* 2018; 99(9): 569–76. https://doi.org/10.1016/j.diii.2018.02.008.

13 Abnormalities of Second Stage

Gowri Dorairajan
Jawaharlal Institute of Postgraduate Medical
Education and Research (JIPMER)

When the second stage is delayed, there might be a dilemma as to how to deliver the woman. Sometimes it is a challenging decision to deliver by assisted methods or by opting for a caesarean section. The second stage is prolonged when it is longer than 2 hours in a primigravida or one 1 hour in a multigravida labouring without regional anaesthesia. An hour is added in a woman receiving epidural analgesia. Irrespective of the time frame, one needs to be alert for overt signs of disproportion once she is in the second stage and make the decision for the mode of delivery accordingly.

A good part of the journey and rotation of the head occurs in the second stage of labour. If features of disproportion become manifest by the end of the passive phase, then active bearing down may be terminated in favour of an emergency caesarean section. The fetal heart rate needs to be monitored continuously by the electronic monitor or every 5 minutes by intermittent auscultation. The woman should never be left alone in the second stage of labour. Adequate time should be given for descent to happen passively. Premature attempts at active bearing down may make an obstetrician impatient and might result in unnecessary operative instrumentation. According to the recent guidelines by the consortium of labour, the second stage can be extended to 3 hours in a primigravida and 2 hours in a multigravida, provided there are no maternal and fetal compromise and there are no signs of disproportion on abdominal or internal examination. Active bearing down as soon as the second stage begins may be necessary if there is the presence of any alerting features and if the head is already at the lower station. Earlier intervention by operative delivery or caesarean delivery may become necessary in some situations with fetal heart rate abnormalities.

At the beginning of the second stage, one must carefully note down the adequacy of uterine activity and the fifths palpable on abdominal examination. In addition, one should carefully assess and note the station, caput, moulding, liquor colour, degree of deflexion, if any, and the adequacy of the lower strait. The notes will help compare with repeat findings more objective, especially when the obstetric caregivers are different in a high turnover labour room with shift duties. In the second stage, due to the strong uterine contractions and reduction in liquor, sometimes it may become difficult to assess the position of the fetus on abdominal examination and caput may obscure the delineation of sutures. Referring to admission notes will help in reaffirming the position. If caput obscures the internal examination findings, then ultrasonography is useful to rule out asynclitism and ascertain the side of the back and the position of the head.

ARREST IN THE SECOND STAGE OF LABOUR

When the second stage is confirmed, active vigilance should start for the descent of the head, fetal heart rate, and any features of cephalo-pelvic disproportion. Depending on the parity, up to half to 1 hour can be allowed for the passive descent of the head and spontaneous urge to push. We need to expedite vaginal delivery by encouraging active bearing down or by operative assistance in the following situations:

> Suspicious fetal heart rate, especially severe early deceleration and variable deceleration suggestive of nuchal cord. In women with pathological CTG pattern.

DOI: 10.1201/9781003034360-13

1. The woman had been in a prolonged active phase of labour.
2. High-risk conditions in women preclude prolonged bearing down such as hypertension, preeclampsia, and heart disease.
3. For women with previous caesarean section, scars are more likely to disrupt in the second stage. Reducing the second stage duration will reduce the exposure of the scarred area to strong uterine contractions.
4. More than 1 hour has passed, and there is no urge to push and in the absence of features suggestive of cephalopelvic disproportion.
5. In women undergoing a trial of labour.

Following are the points in favour of termination by caesarean section if 1 hour of active bearing down does not result in successful delivery, even if the fetal heart rate pattern is reassuring:

a. Fetal poles are still palpable on abdominal examination.
b. The head has not advanced beyond +1 station.
c. There is progressively increasing caput formation.
d. Progressively increasing moulding in more than one suture.
e. Secondary uterine inertia requiring escalating oxytocin infusion.
f. As mentioned earlier, secondary inertia is a protective mechanism in the second stage and alerts about possible subtle disproportion. Quite often, one realizes that if not recognized and terminated by caesarean section, one may achieve vaginal delivery at the cost of either severe birth asphyxia or severe shoulder dystocia or unwarranted and severe trauma to the vulva and vagina. A wrong decision may result in unjustified and unacceptably high maternal morbidity, perinatal morbidity, and even mortality.
g. Poor-fitting of the head with the head at a higher station will be associated with an empty sacral hollow. Higher station precludes instrumental delivery.
h. If the head fits too tight and the vagina around is too dry and or oedematous or bluish, with no space between the head and the vagina. In such a situation, invariably, the poles will be palpable.
i. Presence of severe asynclitism or severe deflexed head (median presentation).
j. Of course, the occurrence of pathological or category III fetal heart rate pattern will compel a caesarean section if it is not amenable to operative vaginal delivery.

Thus, extreme vigilance of evolving findings on the digital vaginal exam and the fetal heart rate pattern is important. Even after achieving the second stage, the obstetrician should keep the options open for termination by caesarean section.

I would like to describe a case.

An otherwise low-risk primigravida was admitted in labour due to premature rupture of membranes at term at 5.30 am. The admitting resident noted a single fetus in ROT position with a clinical estimate of 3 kg with a reassuring fetal heart rate. Clear liquor was draining from the vagina. The uterus was relaxed. The right ischial spine was noted to be slightly prominent. After 4 hours of waiting for spontaneous onset of labour pain, induction was started at 10 am. Regular contractions were achieved, and after 4 hours, the cervix was found to be 5 cm dilated. The position mentioned was left occipito-anterior on digital examination. After 4 hours of good uterine contractions at 5.30 pm also the findings remained the same on digital examination. Since the fetal heart rate was reassuring, the residents decided that the labour could continue. She did not require more than 12 mIU/minute of oxytocin. The contractions were optimum.

Another 4 hours later (9.30 pm), she was 6 cm dilated with full effacement and vertex had descended to −1 station. There was no caput or moulding. At 1.30 am, she was fully dilated. There was a ++ caput and moulding score of 4/6. There was early deceleration observed though the variability was good, and the fetal heart was recovering well in between contractions. The resident waited for an hour for the descent of head. The head reached up to +2 cm station even after active bearing down. The registrar attempted mid cavity forceps delivery. However, the blades could not be inserted, and so a vacuum was applied, and with a second pull, an asphyxiated baby with a poor Apgar score was delivered. The baby was 3 kg and had severe hypoxia.

It was admitted to NICU but died after 5 days due to ischaemic encephalopathy and acidosis. The baby received hypothermic treatment for encephalopathy. There was a subgaleal bleed and encephalomalacia on imaging.

Study the case and

a. Point out the problems and the missed alerting signs.
b. What do you think would be the position of the fetus?
c. How would you have delivered the woman?

Analysis of the above case: The woman was in active labour 4 hours after starting induction. The tardy progress after reaching the active phase of labour is a crucial alerting sign. Despite good uterine contractions, she remained at 5 cm for 4 hours. Reassessment of the position, the pelvis, if needed by a senior, should have been done at this stage.

At the second stage, significant moulding and caput were noted with the head at +1 station. The findings like caput and moulding were noted but were disregarded and not interpreted as signs of frank cephalopelvic disproportion (CPD). The extension of the second stage by another 1 hour was not justified, especially when there was recurrent severe early deceleration observed. That was the next alerting sign that was not interpreted properly. The admitting registrar noted the position as ROT; the subsequent team misjudged the ROP as LOA.

This emphasizes the importance of the first examination at admission. The original findings should be referred to later when the progress is tardy as the original comment on position on clinical examination is more reliable. The case should have been delivered by caesarean section. At least when the woman reached the second stage the signs of disproportion should have been recognized. When the forceps blade did not lock, it was another warning sign, and the operative delivery should have been abandoned in favour of caesarean delivery.

To reemphasize, the goal of labour is not to achieve vaginal birth but to achieve the birth of a baby without asphyxia.

Deep transverse arrest (DTA): Despite good uterine contractions at full dilatation, the head is arrested at zero station with sagittal suture in the transverse diameter of the maternal pelvis and the head fails to descend and deliver after 2 hours, then it is referred to as deep transverse arrest. Typically, this is one of the fates of labour starting in the occipitoposterior position. The transverse arrest can be high that is at "0" station or sometimes low at +1 or +2 station. It is important to anticipate this condition.

Risk factors for deep transverse arrest: The following factors are likely to favour the development of transverse arrest

Borderline mid pelvis or lower strait of the pelvis: Careful assessment of the inter-ischial spine level (plane of least pelvic dimensions) needs to be done in all cases with special focus for women with malposition and in short-statured women.

A persistent deflexed head: If the head fails to flex, then the bigger diameter of the head presents, resulting in relative disproportion.

A big baby: When the clinical estimation is more than 3.5 kg, it is prudent to have a scan estimation. Scan estimation being more accurate will help to flag the case during labour and a quicker decision should be taken to deliver by caesarean in case of tardy progress or malposition and early features of disproportion.

Oligohydramnios: Adequate liquor is necessary for the shoulders to rotate internally.

Caesarean section should be considered as the option in the presence of inadequate mid pelvis. There is no role of a trial of assisted vaginal birth for mid pelvis problems.

MANAGEMENT OF DEEP TRANSVERSE ARREST

When this condition is diagnosed, the following factors will favour delivery by **caesarean section:** Borderline or inadequate mid pelvis and lower strait, big baby, or high station of 0 or +1, signs of CPD like significant moulding and caput, meconium-stained liquor, and pathological fetal heart rate pattern.

In the presence of average size fetus, reassuring fetal heart rate pattern, adequate mid pelvis, and lower strait, the head that is at or below +2 cm station, the options to complete vaginal delivery are as follows:

- Manual rotation and forceps extraction.
- Forceps rotation and extraction.
- Vacuum-assisted delivery.

Manual rotation and forceps extraction

Before carrying out this procedure, the checklist mentioned in Box 13.1 should be ensured.

The woman should be placed in a lithotomy position, and the parts, including the lower abdomen, should be cleaned and draped. The urinary bladder should be emptied, and the position of the head and the back of the fetus should be correctly ascertained clinically and, if needed, substantiating by ultrasound. The woman should be explained and informed about the procedure.

Half Hand Method

The right hand (Figure 13.1a, fingers and upper palm) is introduced in LOT position and left hand for the ROT position towards the posterior parietal bone. The head is gently lifted and rotated towards the pubic symphysis with contractions. The freehand should manoeuvre the shoulder from the abdomen to the opposite side. If there is adequate liquor and the baby weight is average, then the shoulder movement is likely to be successful. As the occiput moves to direct anteriorly or 45° short of rotation, low forceps can be applied to replace the hand and delivery proceeded with. Easy locking of the blades is a sign of successful rotation.

If the shoulder does not move easily, the occiput can be partially rotated to the anterior position. But, the head tends to fall back to the transverse position. In such a situation, the corresponding blade of the forceps may have to be introduced to prevent the head from falling back to the transverse position. The delivery can be completed only if the forceps lock without difficulty.

Full Hand Method

The full hand is used (Figure 13.1b). The right hand is used for the LOT position. The fingers are at the posterior parietal bone, and the thumb is at the anterior parietal bone. The head is firmly gripped and turned to move the occiput towards the pubic symphysis. It is starting with a supinated hand and

---

BOX 13.1   CHECKLIST FOR MANUAL ROTATION AND FORCEPS EXTRACTION

- Full dilation
- Pelvis adequate
- No features of CPD or obstructed labour
- Reassuring fetal heart rate pattern
- No palpable pole or only sinciput is palpable. Station +2 cm or lower
- Experienced and skilled obstetrician
- Position of fetus made out with certainty
- The bladder is empty

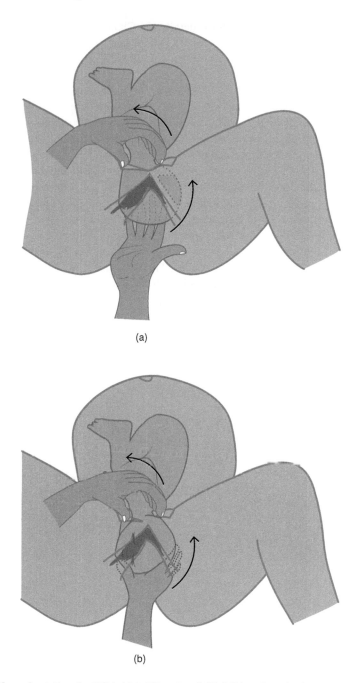

(a)

(b)

FIGURE 13.1 Manual rotation for DTA (a) half hand and (b) full hand method.

ending in pronation. Other hand manipulates the shoulder from the abdomen to the opposite side. This is followed by low forceps application and extraction, as mentioned above.

Forceps rotation and extraction: This can be done only with Kielland forceps. It is no longer done in modern obstetrics. The advantage of Kielland's forceps is that it has a sliding lock. In modern obstetrics, ventouse extraction has replaced forceps rotation, and the caesarean section is considered the safest option for the fetus and the mother when the malrotated head is at a higher station. Kielland's forceps and application are discussed in Chapter 14.

Ventouse rotation and extraction: This is detailed in Chapter15. It is essential to recognize and place the ventouse cup at the flexion point. Rotation should never be attempted by twisting the cup while pulling it after it is applied. Twisting or turning while pulling can cause scalp avulsion injury. The bird metallic cups are preferred for rotation.

Face to pubis delivery (Figure 13.2): This is a situation encountered in the occipitoposterior position. When the occiput rotates posteriorly by 45°, the sinciput comes under the pubic symphysis. The sagittal suture occupies the anteroposterior diameter of the outlet of the maternal pelvis. The position is a direct occipital posterior position. It is usually the fate of a woman with a high inclination or anthropoid pelvis. If the head is well flexed, the sinciput hinges under the pubic symphysis. Suppose it is deflexed. The root of the nose hinges against the pubic symphysis. On internal examination, the sagittal suture is in the midline, and the lambda is felt posteriorly. In the deflexed head or median presentation, the sinciput will be felt easily in the centre of the pelvis. Sometimes it may be exceedingly difficult to appreciate the sutures due to caput formation and prolonged labour. This further emphasizes the need to assess and document the position carefully at admission to the labour room. In the direct occipital posterior position, the wider biparietal diameter is placed posteriorly. The delivery happens as face to pubes. The vertex, followed by the occiput, is born by flexion. This is followed by the birth of the sinciput, forehead, and face by extension. Therefore, at crowning, the direction of head movement is first upwards, then downwards. The same direction should be followed if forceps are applied to deliver the head. Since the wider biparietal diameter is stretching the perineum, the chance of complete perineal tear is very high, and so good perineal support is essential to prevent the same.

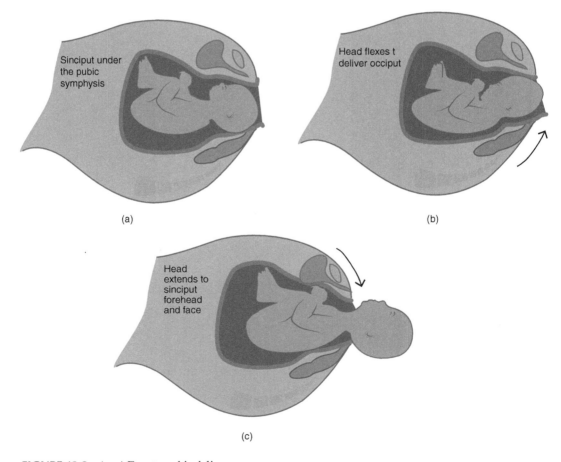

(a)

(b)

(c)

FIGURE 13.2   (a–c) Face to pubis delivery.

OBSTRUCTED LABOUR AND BANDL'S RING

When despite good uterine contractions for 2 hours in the second stage, the labour comes to a standstill due to a mechanical cause, it is called obstructed labour. Thus, the problem lies with the passage or the passenger. It is important to anticipate and have a high index of suspicion for the following situations as the underlying cause of obstructed labour.

- Short-statured primigravida (Contracted pelvis)
- Big baby
- Malpresentation
- Deflexed head
- Malposition
- Brow presentation.

Obstructed labour is more likely to happen in a primigravida. Secondary inertia of the uterus is a protective phenomenon and is likely to be encountered in the above situations as a natural means of preventing obstructed labour and ruptured uterus.

Pathophysiology of Obstructed Labour

In the second stage, the upper segment's strong uterine contractions and retraction result in excessive stretching of the lower segment to 10–15 cm. The upper segment is felt as the shortened, hardened upper part. The junction between the two segments keeps rising and is felt on abdominal examination as a ring that may reach as high as the level of the umbilicus. This pathological ring is called **the Bandl's ring** (Figure 11.1g, Chapter 11).

The urinary bladder also gets stretched and compressed and may become palpable per abdomen along with the lower segment. Because of the obstruction of labour, the urethra-vesical junction gets compressed between the pubic symphysis and the advancing head. The bladder becomes oedematous. The bladder base is subjected to pressure between the advancing head and the pubic bone. The bladder base may eventually necrose to form a vesicovaginal fistula if the second stage gets prolonged and immediate delivery is not done to relieve the compression.

Clinical Features

The woman appears exhausted and dehydrated. There is tachycardia. She may be febrile because of exhaustion and later because of sepsis. There may be ketotic breath with the characteristic smell. The blood pressure, however, remains normal.

Abdominal examination reveals a tense tender uterus and a firmly retracted and tender upper segment. The contractions are extraordinarily strong to begin with, and later secondary inertia of the uterus sets in. The lower segment is stretched and palpable. Bandl's ring is palpated anywhere between the pubic symphysis and the umbilicus. The urinary bladder is full and palpable to a variable extent above the pubic symphysis.

The liquor is drained, and it is nearly impossible to make out the presentation or the position on abdominal examination. Both the poles might be palpable per abdomen. Sometimes distended bowel loops may be seen on the flanks due to distension proximal to the compression of the sigmoid colon between the head and the pelvic bone. The fetal heart sounds are likely to be absent or manifest bradycardia. On digital vaginal examination, the vagina feels dry and warm. In vertex presentation, the head is felt jammed. There is a large pelvic caput and more than 4/6 moulding. There may be asynclitism observed. The caput might obscure the sutures, and it may be difficult to ascertain the position of the head. There may be meconium-stained liquor. One should assess the cause of obstruction like the malposition and the inadequacy of the mid and lower strait of the pelvis. In certain situations, the cervical lips may be felt as oedematous and thickened lips (this may be misperceived as not fully dilated). It is more likely in high obstruction with the presenting part high up or not filling like the transverse lie.

THE FATE OF OBSTRUCTED LABOUR

The full-blown picture described above is no longer observed in the present-day scenario, probably due to earlier detection and prompt caesarean delivery to relieve the obstruction.

A primigravida is more likely to go into obstructed labour. A multigravida may present with a rupture of the uterus. Secondary inertia is a protective phenomenon against rupture and is more likely in a primigravida.

If not recognized and promptly treated, obstructed labour can result in perinatal asphyxia and fetal death. The following are the complications of obstructed labour:

1. Maternal sepsis.
2. Perinatal hypoxia can be worsened by sepsis and meconium aspiration resulting in a neurological sequel if the neonate survives.
3. Rupture of uterus in a multigravida.
4. Postpartum haemorrhage.
5. Operative interference to mother with caesarean section increases her morbidity. There is a higher risk of intraoperative bladder injury while opening the abdomen. There is a risk of tear of the lower segment, broad ligament hematoma formation, and extension of the uterine incision to the vagina as the lower segment is thinned out and friable.
6. Obstetric vesical-vaginal fistula if the obstruction is not promptly relieved.
7. Maternal mortality due to haemorrhage and sepsis.

PREVENTION OF OBSTRUCTED LABOUR

Having a high index of suspicion is necessary. Careful clinical assessment should be done before the onset of labour to rule out inadequate pelvis in a primigravida, especially if she is a short-statured woman.

Careful assessment of the pelvis is also required in women with big babies and malposition. Vigilance for features of CPD when such a woman is in labour will help pick up abnormal findings and avert full-blown obstructed labour.

It is necessary to respect secondary inertia in a primigravida after she has achieved the spontaneous active phase of labour. It is important to carefully reassess the fetal weight, position, and architecture of the pelvis in such women before whipping the uterus with oxytocin augmentation.

In such situations of secondary inertia undergoing augmentation with oxytocin infusion, it is necessary to have continued vigilance, and early decision for caesarean section should be taken if features of caput/ moulding/asynclitism/coning appear.

We should always remember that the goal of the obstetrician should not be to achieve full dilation or vaginal delivery at the cost of severe fetal asphyxia or fetal death. The goal is active vigilance and balance between vaginal delivery and the decision for caesarean section to deliver a healthy neonate.

TREATMENT OF OBSTRUCTED LABOUR

In a full-blown case of obstructed labour, delivery by caesarean section is a wise choice to reduce further morbidity to the woman. In a rare case of intrauterine death, a decision of destructive procedure or operative instrumental delivery in expert hands may save a caesarean section. One must remember that there is a high chance of rupture of the lower segment and its consequences, and so, before embarking on the decision for operative vaginal delivery, impending rupture should be ruled out. Resuscitation of the woman with an intravenous rush of fluids and antibiotics is important and should be carried out parallel to better the woman's recovery. One must recognize that the pre-existing fluid loss due to prolonged second stage, stress, and exhaustion of labour can be enormous. Continuous bladder drainage for 2–3 weeks may be necessary if there was oedema of the bladder and blood-stained urine before the operation to prevent the development of obstetric fistula later.

One must be prepared for atonic as well as traumatic postpartum haemorrhage. The caesarean section for obstructed labour requires extreme caution and is discussed in Chapter 16.

SHOULDER DYSTOCIA

When the shoulders fail to deliver either spontaneously or with gentle traction after the delivery of the head, it is diagnosed as shoulder dystocia. Objectively, if the delivery time between head and shoulder exceeds 60 seconds and requires additional manoeuvres to deliver, it is called shoulder dystocia.

Diagnosis: When the head seems to retract at the perineum without undergoing restitution after the delivery, there is a strong possibility of shoulder dystocia. It is also called a *turtle sign*. Invariably the baby's face reflects macrosomia with chubby cheeks. Sometimes with gentle manipulation or even spontaneously, the restitution might occur, but after that, the second stage comes to a standstill, and the shoulders refuse to deliver. The problem at hand is that the bis-acromion diameter is in the AP diameter of the outlet, and the anterior shoulder is arrested behind and above the pubic symphysis.

Fetal concerns: The time starts ticking from head delivery. The time available from delivery of head to shoulders is 5 minutes to prevent asphyxia. Asphyxia sets in because the cord is getting compressed, and the fetus cannot take a breath on its own.

The next concern is trauma to the fetus like brachial plexus injury or fracture of the humerus and or clavicle.

Fetal death will be the worst scenario if it is not delivered on time.

Don'ts: It is natural for the obstetrician to panic – panic results in a reaction of wrong manoeuvres resulting in more harm to the fetus.

It is important not to give lateral traction (downward or upward) on the fetal head or pulling strongly on the head and neck, resulting in brachial plexus injury.

Do's: Note down the time. Call for help includes an assistant, anaesthetist as standby, and the paediatrician as the baby is likely to be born with a low Apgar score.

Extend the episiotomy or **perform a liberal mediolateral episiotomy**: This will improve the access for performing the manoeuvres and reduce tissue resistance at delivery. But this may not be easy when the head is tightly retracted at the perineum. So liberal anticipatory episiotomy helps in cases with a high index of suspicion.

Ascertain the side where the back is. It is easy to know this by looking for the occiput. Back would be on the same side as where the occiput is.

Ascertain the level of the posterior shoulder: The manoeuvres are based on the level of the posterior shoulder.

Suppose the posterior shoulder is in the pelvis below the level of the ischial spines. In that case, it is the anterior shoulder that is jammed above the pelvic inlet or the pubic symphysis. The manoeuvre used is the **McRoberts manoeuvre** (Figure 13.3a).

McRoberts manoeuvre: This involves lifting the thigh of the woman and hyper-flexing them over her abdomen. Two attendants are needed for the two thighs. This position rotates the pubic symphysis and changes its inclination, thereby allowing the anterior shoulder to slip beneath it. This position also further pushes the coccyx backwards and widens the available anteroposterior diameter of the outlet of the pelvis. This should be supplemented by *suprapubic pressure* by an assistant in a downward lateral direction (from left to right if the back is on the left side) to release the shoulder by pushing obliquely, and the obstetrician should give axial traction from below. The obstetrician can release the anterior shoulder by placing fingers on the posterior aspect of the anterior shoulder and giving pressure to the opposite side (right hand placed at the backside of the anterior shoulder LOT position).

In most situations, this manoeuvre successfully releases and delivers the shoulder.

This manoeuvre is of no use **if the posterior shoulder is high up.**

If the posterior shoulder is high up or if the McRoberts manoeuvre fails to deliver the fetus, then we need to attempt to **deliver the posterior arm** (Figure 13.3b). The hand of the obstetrician corresponding to the ventrum of the fetus (left hand if fetal back is on the left) is introduced till one reaches the cubital fossa. The hand should splint the humerus of the fetus by remaining parallel to the fetal arm, and no attempt should be made to give any tangential pressure on the arm. Gentle pressure on the cubital fossa will flex the elbow and allow grabbing of the hand. The hand is swept across the chest, and the posterior shoulder is delivered out by extending the arm. The delivery of the anterior shoulder follows automatically on gentle traction. If it fails, then the fetus must be rotated by 180 degrees to bring the anterior shoulder towards the sacrum and deliver it.

Fracture of the humerus is a distinct complication and can be reduced by pressure at the elbow and not the arm and by sweeping the fetal hand in the correct direction by adduction across the fetus's chest.

The next manoeuvre when the posterior shoulder is low down is now described (**Rubin I manoeuvr**e). Suprapubic pressure is applied in a downward and lateral direction from the backside of the anterior shoulder towards the fetal face. This step gets the bisacromial diameter from the narrower anteroposterior diameter to the larger oblique diameter of the maternal inlet, which will aid in the delivery of the fetus by gentle axial traction. Sometimes rocking movement instead of steady movement of the shoulder by the abdominal hand may be necessary.

Wood's corkscrew manoeuvre (Figure 13.3c): The posterior shoulder is pushed from anterior to posterior (front to back) direction with the hand of the obstetrician. (The left hand of obstetrician if the back of the fetus is on the left side.) An assistant gives suprapubic pressure with the base of the fisted palm pushing the anterior shoulder in the posterior (backside) to an anterior direction (that means in the direction towards the fetal face). The suprapubic pressure is directed downwards and laterally. There should be good synchronization between the abdominal assistant and the obstetrician at the foot end. The idea is to rotate the shoulder progressively by 180°. This helps to dislodge the anterior shoulder and bring the bisacromial diameter to oblique diameter. Once the anterior shoulder is dislodged from behind the symphysis, it can be delivered by gentle axial traction. If not, the movement is continued to make it rotate further. The posterior shoulder that was within the pelvis comes anteriorly and will be below the pubic symphysis and hence can be delivered easily.

The **reverse Wood's corkscrew**: In this manoeuvre, the concept is to reduce the bisacromial diameter by pushing both the shoulders towards the chest. Suppose the fetal back is on the left side of the mother. In that case, the left hand of the obstetrician is inserted on the backside of the posterior shoulder and the shoulder is pushed towards the chest to reduce the bisacromial diameter. This step aided with axial traction would deliver the shoulders.

Placing the women in **an all-four position** followed by downward traction on the posterior shoulder (the one towards the maternal sacrum) can be attempted (Gaskin manoeuvre). However, it may not be logistically possible as many personnel are needed to change the position, and an exhausted mother may not be able to assume the position voluntarily.

If nothing works and the posterior shoulder is held above the brim, then the last resort would be to reposit the head and perform a caesarean section. Repositing the head may be difficult.

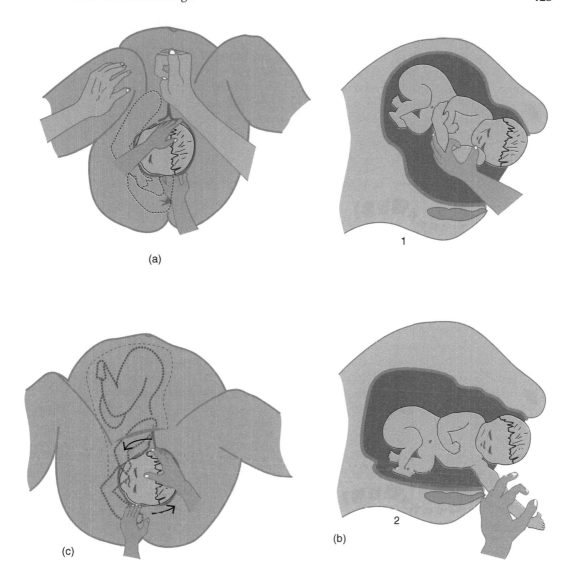

(a)

1

(c)

2

(b)

FIGURE 13.3 Management of shoulder dystocia: (a) McRoberts manoeuvre; (b) bringing the hand down; and (c) Wood's corkscrew method.

It involves reverse steps, which means rotate back the sagittal suture to the midline and flex the head and reposition in the vagina while traction is being given on the baby during cae-sarean section from the uterine incision to extract the baby. This is also called the **Zavanelli manoeuvr**e.

Cleidotomy is the last resort to deliver the baby vaginally after deliberately fracturing the clavi-cle of the fetus with strong pressure on the anterior clavicle. It can be attended by injury to the sub-clavian vessels. The fracture of the clavicle heals well. **Symphysiotomy** is a very morbid procedure and may have long-term problems and has no role in modern obstetrics. **Abdominal rescue** can be done without repositing the head. A lower segment uterine incision followed by a rotation of the shoulder to oblique diameter by directly working on the shoulder can help complete the delivery from the vaginal end. This can be attempted if the fetus is still alive.

COMPLICATIONS OF SHOULDER DYSTOCIA

Fetal: As already mentioned, there can be brachial plexus injury, fractures of the humerus and the clavicle, birth asphyxia, and fetal death. Fetal bruising due to handling can also occur.

Maternal complications: Increased operative interference, an extension of episiotomy, tears in the vagina, complete perineal tear, cervical tear, rupture of the uterus, postpartum haemorrhage, and sepsis, especially when a caesarean section is resorted to.

PREVENTION OF SHOULDER DYSTOCIA

A high index of suspicion and anticipation is necessary. The following risk factors should be looked out for:

a. **Diabetes with macrosomia**: Fetuses of diabetic women have a tendency to accumulate fat around the shoulder and the abdominal wall. Estimated weight above 4.5 kg in a woman with diabetes should be delivered by prelabour scheduled caesarean section. We take a cut-off of 4 kg fetal weight in a woman with diabetes for deciding for caesarean section in our hospital.

b. **Previous history of shoulder dystocia**: The recurrence risk is high. The previous history should alert us for careful assessment of the baby's weight and the architecture of the pelvis in the index pregnancy.

c. **Multiparity**: The fetal weight increases in subsequent pregnancies. The fact that the woman has previously delivered a good size baby might make us take our guard off. But a slightly bigger baby could result in shoulder dystocia in the index pregnancy.

d. Tardy progress of labour, incoordinate uterine contraction, or secondary inertia is a forewarning alert.

A difficult instrumental delivery might deliver the head, but the shoulders might get trapped. So, if the expected fetal weight is on the higher side and the second stage is prolonged, one could still decide for caesarean section instead of difficult instrumental delivery.

DELIVERING MULTIPLE PREGNANCIES

The second stage in multiple pregnancies poses peculiar problems and requires vigilance. There is no role of a trial of vaginal delivery in monoamniotic-monochorionic twins.

If the first is a non-vertex presentation, it is prudent to consider a prelabour caesarean section.

In situations where the first twin is vertex and the second twin is non-vertex, many hospitals may still consider caesarean section. The morbidity of the second twin is always higher due to problems of malpresentation, cord prolapse, abruption, and increased operator interference for its delivery. The decision for the mode of delivery with only the second one in non-vertex presentation rests on many factors such as the period of gestation, the discordance of weight, chorionicity, type of conception, and age of the woman. In our centre and many developing countries where salvageability below 30 weeks of gestation is around 60%, vagina delivery is encouraged, especially if labour is spontaneous and conception was not an issue. Even among those with both vertexes, the second twin presentation can change to transverse lie or breech after delivering the first twin.

So, let us discuss the diamniotic twins, with the first presenting as a vertex. It is expected that the first twin should deliver uneventfully. However, there can be tardy progress of labour due to over-distention compounded by polyhydramnios. The labour might need augmentation with oxytocin. It is prudent to ensure intravenous access. Blood should be cross-matched and kept ready in case of need for operating intervention or third-stage complication. At the second stage, the delivery of first vertex is usually uneventful and spontaneous. The twins are likely to be only average birth weight. In the case of prematurity, an episiotomy should be considered to prevent compression of the head. One should avoid sudden decompression of the head at birth. So the head should be delivered slowly. Once the first twin is delivered, the cord is clamped with two clamps and cut in between so that one clamp remains at the fetal end. Then one should do a vagina examination for the presenting part as well as the status of the cervix. If the second twin is also vertex, an artificial rupture of membranes can be done once the head fixes. The cervix might often retract, and the uterine contractions may become lesser in intensity after the first twin is delivered. Therefore, it is prudent to accelerate the power of the uterine contractions with a low dose of oxytocin infusion. Once the contractions resume in good intensity, the vertex descends and we can anticipate uneventful birth.

If after the delivery of the first twin, a tense bag appears to distend the vagina, please do not poke to feel the presenting part; instead, perform an abdominal examination to ascertain the presentation and to note the fetal heart sounds.

If the second twin is in a transverse lie, it is worthy of performing an external cephalic or external podalic version with a preference for an external cephalic version. If it is breech, then one needs to ascertain the type of breech and wait for its descent. The membranes can be preserved till the presenting part descends with contractions to prevent cord prolapse. Once a longitudinal lie is achieved and contractions have been re-established, one can proceed with controlled artificial rupture of membranes and anticipate descent of the presenting part. Spontaneous vaginal delivery can be completed for the vertex presentation. In the case of breech, assisted breech delivery must be conducted once climbing occurs. If the breech fails to deliver spontaneously after descending into the pelvis, then extraction might be necessary.

If, however, the external version fails, then an internal podalic version (IPV) can be attempted. IPV should be done only under anaesthesia, preferably general anaesthesia in the operation theatre. There should be backup and full preparation for emergency caesarean section/laparotomy readily available.

Internal Podalic Version

In the operation theatre, the patient is put in the dorsal lithotomy position. The vulva, thigh, and abdomen should be cleaned and draped. It is vital to know the baby's exact position inside the uterus before attempting an IPV. We should know the position of the back, the head, and the lower limbs to ensure that the feet are held and pulled out, and the hand should not be confused with the feet. So, under anaesthesia, the vaginal examination is repeated. The membranes are ruptured if intact. The right hand is introduced inside the vagina. The hand is introduced up to the fundus to feel and hold the feet of the baby firmly and bring it down. In dorsoinferior and dorsoanterior positions, one may have to go all the way above and beyond the trunk of the fetus to reach the feet. Sometimes deepening of anaesthesia is mandated when the liquor has flowed out already. After bringing the feet down, breech extraction is done to deliver the fetus. As soon as the fetus is born, the anaesthetist should be informed to lighten the plane of anaesthesia so that the uterus can resume back contractions. Placental removal should be attempted after uterine contractions resume and after ensuring signs of placental separation. Manual removal of the placenta is not necessary as it may be attended by significant bleeding. After placental delivery, the uterus needs to be palpated from the abdomen and by the vaginal hand to ensure it is well contracted and not ruptured. In the event of continued excessive bleeding and suspected rupture of the uterus or tear of the cervix, a suitable exploration of the cervix or, if need be, laparotomy may be necessary to tackle the trauma to the reproductive tract.

In the event of significant abruption with retracted collapse cervix or spontaneous rupture of the membrane with cord prolapse or fetal heart rate abnormality with collapsed cervix/high up presenting part or transverse lie with the collapsed cervix and drained liquor, a caesarean section may become necessary to deliver the second twin. The cord should be cut between three clamps leaving two clamps towards the fetal side. This is to make the distinction that the cord belongs to the second twin. The number of clamps towards the umbilical cord can correspond to the order of the fetus in higher order multiple gestations,

Colour coding of the clamps can help delineate which placenta belongs to which fetus and know the chorionicity between the various fetuses. The time difference recorded between the delivery of the twins is variable. The shortest of 22.976 seconds (on the 6th April 2017 in Canada) and the longest of 153 days [1] has been recorded. There is no cut-off for the upper limit of the inter-twin delivery duration. However, longer than half an hour increases the adverse outcomes of twin two and one needs to expedite the delivery. One needs to assess for the cause for delay in the second stage to decide on appropriate intervention.

Abruption, cord prolapse, malpresentation, increased operative intervention, delayed delivery, and difficult delivery are the reasons for adverse perinatal morbidity and mortality for the second twin in comparison to the first twin.

REFERENCE

Hamersley SL, Coleman SK, Bergauer NK, Bartholomew LM, Pinckert TL. Delayed-interval delivery in twin pregnancies. *J Reprod Med.* 2002; 47: 125–130.

14 Forceps Delivery

Gowri Dorairajan
Jawaharlal Institute of Postgraduate Medical
Education and Research (JIPMER)

When completing vaginal delivery requires assistance with some instrumentation, it is called operative or assisted vaginal delivery. It includes forceps- and vacuum-assisted extraction.

Vaginal delivery assisted by forceps is an art and a great asset to complete vaginal delivery in certain situations. Started by the family of Chamberlain, the forceps have undergone a lot of modifications. There is a limited but definite and irreplaceable role of forceps in modern obstetrics. The rotational Kielland forceps (Figure 14.1a) has slowly become obsolete.

We will discuss forceps by knowing their types and parts.

PARTS OF THE FORCEPS

Forceps are a pair (two branches) of instruments invariably made of metal (Figure 14.1b). The following are the parts of each branch of the forceps:

- Blade
- Shank
- Handle

Blade: The blade has toes and heel. Toes are the ones in the pelvis, and the heel is where it continues as the shank. These are the metallic part which holds the head. They were earlier solid but now are available as fenestrated. Fenestration improves the grip on the fetal head and also makes it lightweight. The blades have a cephalic curve towards the left or right to hold the fetal head. In addition, they have a pelvic curve along their margin to fit along the curve of the pelvis and the perineum, respectively. The one with the minor pelvic curve is the Kielland and Barton forceps. These have maximum flexibility and are used for rotating the head. The one with a reverse pelvis curve (Pipers forceps) is useful for the aftercoming head. These have pronounced reverse curves to accommodate and allow resting on the perineum (reverse pelvic curve).

Shank: The shank is the part that connects the blades to the handle. It could be either long (e.g. Simpson's low forceps and mid cavity forceps) or short (outlet forceps). In addition, the shanks could be parallel to each other (e.g. Simpsons forceps) or cross each other (e.g. Elliot's forceps). When the shanks are parallel and overlap (e.g. Kielland forceps), the perineum is less likely to be stretched than those with parallel left and right shanks set at a distance once the pair is assembled. This fact is extremely useful in understanding the design of rotational forceps.

Handles: The handles of the branches are the ones that allow grip to the obstetricians. They can be plain and smooth or grooved for better grip. Some have an outward projection (Shoulders) towards the outer aspect to prevent slippage of the grip during traction.

It is essential to understand that the branches always cross. In other words, the handle set to the right side will correspond to the blade set on the left side and vice versa. This is designed to form a cup between the two cephalic curves to hold the head. This also makes it easy to understand that the operator's right hands hold the handle of the branch that is applied to the right side of the pelvis of the labouring woman and vice versa.

DOI: 10.1201/9781003034360-14

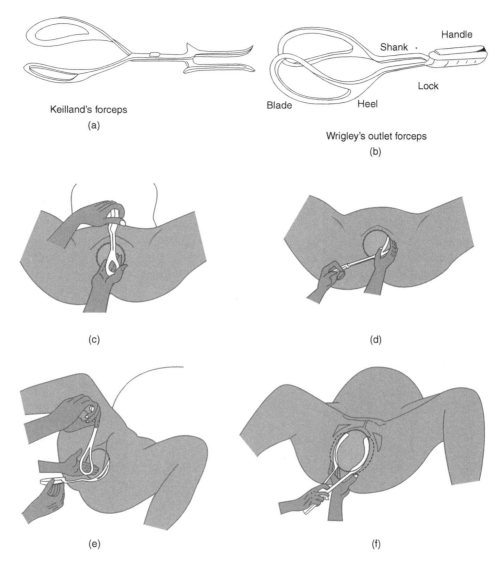

FIGURE 14.1 (a) Kielland forceps. (b) Wrigley's outlet forceps. (c) and (d) Application of the left blade. (e) Application of the right blade as the left blade is held by the assistant. (f) Locking and traction of forceps and perineal support.

It is also important to appreciate that the higher the station, the longer the depth from the vaginal introitus. Therefore, we need forceps with longer shank to deliver the fetus from higher stations (low forceps and mid cavity forceps).

Lock: The lock is an integral part of the forceps to hold the two branches firmly together while applying traction. It is usually at the site of the crossing of the branches. The lock can be of the following types:

a. French lock is a screw system. For example, the Millen Murray mid cavity forceps.
b. English lock as seen in the Wrigley's outlet forceps. It is a double slot lock.
c. The sliding lock, for example, the Kielland forceps lock (Figure 14.1a). The sliding lock permits ease of locking and removal by the sliding mechanism and facilitates double application as may be necessary for rotation and extraction of the head in transverse arrest.

MECHANISM OF WORK OF FORCEPS

1. Compression of the head
2. Rotation of the head
3. Extraction of the head by traction

Depending on the head station, the depth of application and the type of forceps used varies. It can be

1. Mid cavity forceps from 0 to +2 cm station
2. Low forceps: from +2cm to +4 cm station
3. Outlet forceps: from +4 to +5 cm station

THE DIRECTION (AXIS) OF PULL

The direction of pull of the head must correspond with the 'J'-shaped curve of Carus. The direction changes depending on the depth of the forceps application. Therefore, in the higher stations, the pull is downwards. After that, it is outwards, and once it reaches the perineum, the direction changes upwards in the occipito-anterior position. The position of the occiput also governs the direction. The principle of traction is to keep the head well flexed till it reaches the perineum, and once the occiput is delivered, then the direction of traction changes to deliver the rest of the head by extension. So, in direct occipito-posterior position (face to pubes delivery), the traction is outwards and upwards, and after occiput is delivered, the direction changes to downwards.

In the higher station application, the downward pull can be aided by an axis traction device. The axis traction device can be at the heel of blades or shank or the handles (Bill's axis traction). The axis traction at the heels of the blade are bars that fit into a grove at the junction of the blade and the shank. These are fitted to a traction bar (Millen Murrays mid cavity forceps). Pagot Saxtorph's manoeuvre can also achieve downward traction. In this manoeuvre, the operator's left hand is on the shank and applies downward force while traction is used on the handles by the right hand.

PREREQUISITES FOR FORCEPS APPLICATION

A. **Full dilation**: The uterus, cervix, and vagina should have merged to form the birth canal; otherwise forceps blades can cause trauma to the cervix. In other words, the cervix should be fully dilated (not palpable anymore).

B. **Full rotation**: The sagittal suture of the fetal skull should be in the anteroposterior diameter of the outlet of the maternal pelvis. That means the position should be either direct occipito-anterior or direct occipito-posterior position. Forceps can be applied even when the head is 45° short of rotation. Malrotation beyond 45° and occipito-transverse arrest requires either manual or forceps rotation or vacuum extraction. Forceps rotation and extraction are possible with special forceps like the Kiellands or the Barton forceps.

C. The membranes should have been ruptured.

D. *The lower strait of the pelvis should be adequate.* It is important to carefully assess the pelvis and rule out cephalopelvic disproportion features before considering operative instrumental delivery. The application may be complex with elements of disproportion, and there may be difficulty encountered in locking. In such a situation, the traction may not result in successful delivery. If we succeed in delivering, there is a high likelihood of asphyxiated neonate and maternal soft tissue injury.

E. **Station of the head**: The head should be engaged. In modern-day obstetrics, there is no role of forceps extraction for a station above +2 cm station. The various guidelines for forceps application classify the application into:

Mid: 0 to +2 cm station.

Low: below +2 cm but not at the perineum

Outlet: when the head is at the perineum and is visible without retracting the labia

F. The *urinary bladder should be empty.*

G. **Adequate analgesia**: Pudendal block relaxes the pelvic floor. Skin infiltration is necessary before making episiotomy [1]. Local perineal infiltration done for episiotomy might suffice for outlet forceps extraction. Parenteral diazepam, epidural, spinal, paracervical block, and perineal infiltration have been tried, and there is inadequate evidence to support one in favour of the other [2].

H. It is *essential to inform the woman* before the procedure. It is not mandatory to obtain written consent. However, telling her and taking her into confidence is necessary.

TYPES OF APPLICATION

Cephalic application: The blades are applied to fit the head in the mento-vertical diameter. This application reduces the trauma to the eyes and face of the fetus.

Pelvic application: This application is made when the blades are applied along the pelvic sidewalls. Therefore, it is irrespective of the position of the head.

The two applications are the same when the head is fully rotated (occipito-anterior or direct occipito-posterior position).

Indications of forceps application

There are many indications for forceps delivery. The four broad groups are:

1. To expedite delivery when there is a *pathological cardiotocograph.*
2. *Maternal exhaustion/prolonged second stage* or prolonged active phase of the second stage. It is important to be aware of occult cephalopelvic disproportion as the cause of maternal exhaustion. Reassessment of every such prolonged second stage to rule out features of CPD is mandatory before forceps application.
3. *Prophylactic application*: This is to cut short the second stage when we do not want the woman to bear down or Valsalva as it might be harmful to her. Severe preeclampsia, eclampsia, and heart disease are a few examples. It should be kept in mind that all prerequisites for forceps delivery should be met with even for this indication.
4. *Trial of forceps*, When we apply forceps in a borderline disproportion and are aware that there is a likelihood of failure, it is called trial forceps. The fetal condition should be extremely reassuring, and fetal heart rate pattern should be reassuring. The final goal of bringing out a non-asphyxiated neonate with the safety of the maternal tract should always be upheld. So, one should have an open mind to proceed with the caesarean section if the trial fails. The procedure should be abandoned if there is a problem in locking the blades or delivery fails to occur after three pulls. A trial of forceps can be attempted in the operation theatre itself.

Before forceps application, it is important to take verbal consent as already mentioned. However, in cases where prophylactic forceps might be necessary, one can take a more formal documented consent early in labour.

THE PROCEDURE

It should be done under all aseptic precautions.

First and foremost, ensure that the prerequisites are fulfilled.

It is also essential to be aware of the correct position of the fetus. If need be, one must refer to the admission notes because caput may mask the findings at the second stage. Intrapartum ultrasound can be used [3] to confirm in case of any confusion. Misjudging the position and pulling in the wrong direction can fail the procedure or can cause trauma to the mother and asphyxia to the fetus. In my experience, if there is confusion about the position in the second stage, then one must refer to the last antenatal check-up findings and the early labour clinical findings as they are usually more accurate.

One should perform an abdominal examination to ensure that no pole is palpable. In a shallow pelvis, the sinciput may be palpable 1/5th above the pubic symphysis.

On vaginal examination, the sacral follow should be full for all forceps application. The forceps delivery should not be attempted if the sacral hollow is empty.

We must ensure that the vertex and not the caput are at the given station.

Empty the bladder with a red rubber catheter before applying forceps. Phantom application of the forceps (articulation of the branches of the forceps outside) is made outside. The toes of the blade are well lubricated with obstetric cream. Lubricate the vagina with antiseptic obstetric cream. The left branch is applied first. The branch is held by holding the handle vertical (perpendicular to the floor) in the operator's left hand and introduced into the vagina from the midline posteriorly under the guidance of the right hand (Figure 14.1c and d). The fingers of the right hand are between the posterior wall of the vagina and the head. The thumb is at the heel of the blade. The branch is gently slid to the left side of the maternal pelvis with force generated by the right thumb at the heel of the branch. The left hand holding the branch should passively follow without using any force. An assistant then holds it. With a similar manoeuvre, the right branch is introduced by the right hand under the guidance of the left hand (Figure 14.1e). This description is the cephalic application for a fully rotated/45° short of rotation head. The handles are now locked. Generally, the left branch is applied first. In rare situations of ROP position or asynclitism, the right blade can be applied first, but then the locking would require that the left branch should be brought below the right branch. Infiltration of the skin for episiotomy can be done now, if not done, before applying the blades.

Episiotomy: Operative instrumental delivery is an indication for episiotomy. In our hospital, it is made for every operative vaginal delivery. It is usually done after the application of the branches and when crowning occurs with pull. It can also be done before application. This would give more space; however, the bleeding also increases.

Signs of correct application

- Ease of application without force.
- The whole branch has gone in and the heel of the blade is not visible. One should be able to insert only a fingertip, if at all, at the palpable fenestration at the heel of either blade.
- The posterior fontanelle in a fully rotated OA position should be one fingerbreadth above the level of the shanks.
- The blades lock easily.
- When correctly applied, the blades are equidistant from the sagittal suture. And the sagittal suture should be perpendicular to the shanks to ensure that no branch is on the brow or the mastoid region of either side of the fetus and thus, reduces possible neurological and eye trauma.

If the fetus is 45° short of rotation (LOA or ROA) then after locking, the handles should be rotated gently clockwise direction for ROA and anticlockwise for LOA while giving traction to bring it to direct OA position. Otherwise, the toes of the blade might cause pocket tears in the vagina as the forceps are pulled.

Do's and Don'ts about pull

1. Pull only during contractions but deliver the head in between contractions.
2. Pull in the direction along the curve of Carus depending on the station. In this regard, in a higher station, the downward traction can be achieved by the Pajots manoeuvre or by the axis traction at the blades or the shank of the handle, depending on the type of forceps.

3. Pull seated on a chair or height-adjustable stool to ensure limited force generated by the wrist and forearm of one hand of the operator. The arm should be rested with the elbow of the operator resting by the body side. At no cost should the pull be more than that generated by a single operator with one hand on the handles in a standing position with the leg of the operator pressing against the labour table. The other hand of the operator should be supporting the perineum. The pull generated should not be more than 14 kg (30–35 pounds) [4,5].

Perineal support (Figure 14.1f)

Trauma to the perineum and complete perineal tears are serious threats during instrumental deliveries. Complete perineal tears can be drastically reduced by making episiotomy at an angle of 60° from the midline at the time of crowning [4]. The other tip is that during perineal support, instead of stretching the perineum with the left hand, the operator should bunch the skin and sphincter with the finger and thumb of the left hand. After the head is delivered out, the branches are unlocked and removed by reverse movements of each branch so that the handle once again becomes perpendicular to the floor just before removal. Active management of the third stage is performed (Chapter 18). It is mandatory to explore the genital tract thoroughly and also by doing per rectal examination for ruling out any complications to the genital tract such as

- Extension of episiotomy.
- Spiral/pocket-type vaginal tears.
- Cervical tear (described in Chapter 18).
- Complete perineal tear.
- One should be vigilant against traumatic as well as atonic postpartum haemorrhage (PPH). Therefore, all the tears should be promptly sutured.
- Perinatal complications in the form of birth asphyxia, injury to the eyes or facial nerve, galeal or intracranial bleed, and even stillbirth are likely in misjudged and wrong applications of forceps.

Failed forceps

1. Failure to achieve proper locking.
2. Inability to apply correctly on two attempts.
3. Failure of three pulls to achieve descent of the fetus (maximum force generated not to exceed 45 pounds in a primigravida).
4. Slippage of forceps while pulling is likely to happen when the forceps are not correctly applied and there is a lot of gap between the head and the heel of the blade. Slippage on two occasions should alert us that the head is at a higher station and prompt us to abandon the procedure in favour of a caesarean section.
5. The forceps fail if there was a misjudgement of the station due to large caput/missed cephalopelvic disproportion/uncorrected asynclitism.
6. Misjudged position and wrong direction of pull also result in failure and tears to the genital tract.

Key points – Checklist before forceps:

- Check the indication.
- Prerequisites are fulfilled.
- No pole is palpable on abdominal examination.
- Sacral hollow is full.
- Pelvis is adequate.
- Counselling and consent.

- No features of CPD.
- Backup plan available if it fails.

FORCEPS ROTATION AND EXTRACTION

When the sagittal suture is in the transverse diameter of the maternal outlet, the conventional forceps cannot be used. In such a situation, one must use the forceps meant for rotation and extraction.

Kielland forceps: The shanks overlap parallel, and as described earlier, the blades have a minimal pelvic curve. The lack of pelvic curve helps in rotating the head. The presence of a sliding lock makes the removal and reinsertion for extraction very convenient. Lack of pelvic curve makes traction in the direction of the curve of Carus at higher stations easily possible.

For rotation, the forceps can be applied in the classical also called the wandering method.

Classical application (wandering method): Phantom application is made outside. The right blade is anterior in LOT position. The knob faces the occiput. The anterior blade (actually the right blade in LOT position) is applied first under the guidance of the left hand in a manner such as conventional forceps. The direction of the shank at the starting of insertion is at an angle of 45° to the ground. It is then gradually raised to make the shank parallel to the ground. With the thumb of the left hand at the figure guard and counter traction on the shank and handle by the right hand, the blade is moved and applied under the pubic symphysis over the side of the face. The left blade is applied like the conventional forceps from the right side of the vagina under the guiding right hand to slip it posteriorly over the side of the face. The posterior blade can also be applied directly into the sacral hollow from the right side. We must ensure that the shanks don't cross. The finger guard is pulled back to align it and lock it with the anterior blade. This can also correct the asynclitism. The handles are directed downwards then upwards to disimpact the head. The handle now resting parallel to the ground is rotated with figure tip pressure only at the level of handle and shank. After that, traction is carried out to follow the curve of Carus to deliver the fetus.

Direct application: Here the anterior blade is directly applied under the pubis symphysis. The handles are at the level of the bed and gradually raised and brought parallel to the ground. The rest of the procedure is similar to the above technique.

Forceps rotation is associated with severe maternal injuries, including rupture uterus if applied by unskilled hands. It should be attempted under anaesthesia in the operation theatre and should not be attempted if the operator is not trained or skilled in the procedure. There is no role of forceps rotation at higher stations, and this has been replaced with ventouse rotation in the lower stations in modern obstetrics.

REFERENCES

1. Murphy DJ, Strachan BK, Bahl, R on behalf of the Royal College of Obstetricians and Gynaecologists. Assisted vaginal birth. Green-top guideline No. 26. *BJOG.* 2020;127(9):e70–e112. https://doi.org/10.1111/1471-0528.16092.
2. Nikpoor P, Bain E. Analgesia for forceps delivery. *Cochrane Database Syst. Rev.* 2013;(9). Art. No.:CD008878. doi:10.1002/14651858.CD008878.pub2.
3. Ramphul M, Ooi PV, Burke G, Kennelly MM, Said SAT, Montgomery AA, Murphy DJ. Instrumental delivery and ultrasound: a multicentre randomised controlled trial of ultrasound assessment of the fetal head position versus standard care as an approach to prevent morbidity at instrumental delivery. *BJOG.* 2014;121(8):1029–1038.
4. Dennen EH, Dennen PC. *Dennen's forceps deliveries.* 3rd ed. Philadelphia (PA): F.A. Davis; 1989. p. 201.
5. Leslie KK. Dipasquale-Lehnerz P, Smith, M. Obstetric forceps training using visual feedback and the isometric strength testing unit. *Obstet Gynecol.* 2005;105(2):377–382. doi:10.1097/01.AOG.0000150558.27377.a3.

15 Ventouse Delivery

Gowri Dorairajan
Jawaharlal Institute of Postgraduate Medical
Education and Research (JIPMER)

This is a type of assisted vaginal delivery. It is based on the principle of suction force on the fetal head for traction and extraction. This method also achieves automatic rotation if applied correctly. The first such device was invented by Malmstrom in 1953.

An important point to understand is that ventouse or vacuum works well only when applied to the flexion point. In other words, the cup to create the vacuum should be placed over the flexion point.

THE APPARATUS FOR VENTOUSE DELIVERY

The vacuum-assisted birth device has the following parts (Figure 15.1a and b):

- The vacuum cups.
- The suction tubing.
- The traction chain and handle.
- The vacuum creation device.
- Let us understand these in detail.

TYPES OF VENTOUSE CUP

Metal cup: It is available in various sizes from 4 to 6 cm in diameter. The principle of the cup is that the largest diameter is not at the outer rim of the cup but inset by 8 mm from the outer rim (mushroom shape). This is an important principle in the formation of Chignon. Chignon is nothing but oedema of the scalp created by the suction, which is firmly held in the segment between the narrower rim and the widest inset diameter. The metal cup is rigid.

The metal cup has a chain attached to the centre of the convex surface, which can be attached to a traction handle.

The original cup designed by Malmstrom had both the traction device and the suction port at the same place in the centre of the convex surface. Bird modified it by separating the traction hook attachment from the vacuum creation port.

The Bird metal cups are of two types.

The vacuum port where the suction tube is attached can be either on the side (*Bird posterior cup*) (Figure 15.1d) or the convex surface on the side (*Bird anterior cup*) (Figure 15.1a).

The metal cup has a mesh in the concave area to minimize scalp injuries.

The silastic cup: This cup is made of soft silicone material; it is funnel- or bell-shaped with the suction and traction handle at the apex of the funnel (Malmstrom type). It is softer, pliable, and hence, less traumatic.

Kiwi cups (Figure 15.1b inset): These are low profile cups made of silastic material resembling the metal type. Some of these may have a soft sponge in the concave area to further protect the fetus's scalp.

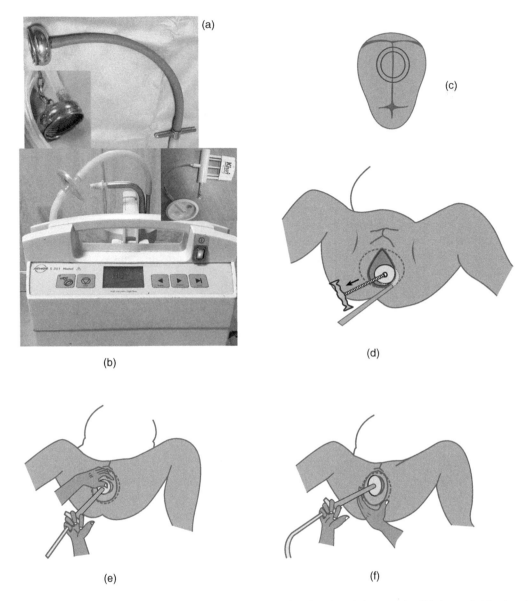

FIGURE 15.1 (a) Photos of the Malmstrom (green suction hose) and the anterior Bird cup (white hose). (b) Photos of the suction device and the inset shows a handheld KIWI system. (c) Line diagram showing the flexion point. (d) Line diagram showing the application of posterior Bird cup for ROP position. (e) Application of Malmstrom cup in an OA position, and position of the left hand while applying traction. (f) Perineal support when the head is at perineum with the left hand.

SUCTION TUBING

This is a transparent or opaque rubber tubing. The traction wire is inside the tubing in the Malmstrom type of cup. The suction tubing in the silastic cup is the thick corrugated tapering end of the funnel type of cup. In the kiwi cup, the suction tubing and the traction wire inside it are very thin and fit into a groove on the concave side of the cup.

It consists of a glass bottle attached to a vacuum extractor or aspirator machine. Usually, these are electrically operated. An aneroid-type dial or a digital monitor (Figure 15.1b) indicates the vacuum generated. In low resource settings, manually operated piston-type devices are used as alternatives. The Kiwi-omni cup device has a handheld pump vacuum device with a vacuum indicator coloured green to red. It also has a traction force indicator.

MECHANISM OF VACUUM ASSISTANCE

The vacuum assists birth in the following ways:

- Improves flexion
- Extraction by traction
- Rotation of the head

Principals of vacuum delivery:

1. The *metal cups* work in the principle of producing chignon, which is scalp oedema generated by slow suction. The widest part of the cup not being at the outer rim gives a firm entrapment of the chignon to allow steady traction.
2. The *silastic cup* does not form a chignon. Here, the cup being silastic gets held onto the scalp by a firm vacuum created at the interface of the scalp and the cup.
3. The most important principle is that the cup should be applied at the flexion point.
4. *Flexion point* (Figure 15.1c) is a point at the midline on the sagittal suture 3 cm in front of the lambda or 6 cm behind the bregma. Traction on this point flexes the head as it descends along the curve of Carus. If wrongly applied, the head will start extending and get stuck or the vacuum cup will slip. In the occipitotransverse position, the cup is in the middle of the vagina, closer to the occipital side. The cup should be applied in the vagina much posterior in the occipitoposterior position as the flexion point is far posterior.
5. The Malmstrom-like cup should not be used for rotation.
6. The posterior type of Bird cup is preferred for rotation of ROP position.
7. Vacuum extraction has to be synchronized with maternal efforts. So, the vacuum traction is applied at the peak of a contraction with maternal efforts.
8. The rotation should never be deliberately done with the cup. That means we should not twist or rotate the traction rod as we pull. Twisting rotational force can cause spiral avulsion of the scalp.
9. With metal cups, the vacuum pressure should be raised gradually over 2 minutes starting from 0.2 kg/cm^2 to 0.8 kg/cm^2 to allow the chignon to form. Whereas, with the silastic cup, it can be immediately raised to 0.8 kg/cm^2.
10. The traction force should always be perpendicular to the cup. Lateral or rocking movement or rotational movement will result in cup detachment and/or scalp avulsion.

Indications:

a. The vacuum device is used in the following situations:
   - Maternal exhaustion
   - Fetal heart rate abnormality
   - Malrotated head including deep transverse arrest
b. It can be used even though a not completely dilated cervix. The cervix should be at least 8 cm dilated.

Contraindications

    a. Vacuum extraction requires maternal efforts of pushing, so it should not be used as prophylactic assistance to avoid Valsalva.

    b. It cannot be used for face presentation.

    c. It should be avoided in the presence of large caput.

    d. It should be avoided in the face to pubes delivery.

    e. Inadequate pelvis, unengaged head, and cephalopelvic disproportion are contraindications.

    f. **Prematurity**: There is a higher risk of intraventricular haemorrhage and scalp injury with vacuum extraction.

    g. **Women on anticoagulants**: Neonates of such women have a higher risk of intracranial bleed with vacuum extraction.

Prerequisites: Like forceps-assisted birth, vacuum assistance should be applied at full dilation though it can be applied even when a rim of the cervix is palpable in dire situations. The head should be engaged and preferably at +2 cm station or below. The membrane should have been ruptured. The exact position of the occiput should be accurately ascertained. The urinary bladder of the women should be emptied. There should be no features of cephalopevic disproportion like severe asynclitism/caput/moulding. The pelvis should be adequate.

APPLICATION AND PULL

Application: Once the indication arises and the perquisites are fulfilled. The women should be counselled, and verbal consent should be obtained.

It is particularly important to be sure about the position of the fetus and hence the side of the occiput to determine the flexion point accurately. In addition, one should check the extractor circuit for adequate suction power before starting.

After cleaning and draping, the outer convex surface of the cup is lubricated with an obstetric cream. The cup is introduced into the vagina. The correct choice of cup is mentioned above and varies depending on the purpose. Posterior metal cups only should be used for rotation of ROP. The cup has to be placed on the flexion point. In rotated head and occipitotransverse position, it will be roughly in the centre of the vagina towards the lambda. In the occipitoposterior position, the cup is likely to be far posteriorly placed (Figure 15.1d). The silastic cup can be folded while inserting into the vagina.

After placing the cup, the fingers of the obstetrician should check along the full circle of the rim of the cup to rule out entrapment of maternal soft tissue like the vagina or the cervix.

One should now start creating the negative vacuum pressure. Once again, after the suction is created, one should double-check with fingers to rule out entrapment of soft tissue. Then the suction pressure is raised as described earlier, either rapidly as in the case of silastic cup or slowly in cases of metal cup till 0.8 cm/kg^2 is achieved. In the kiwi cup with hand-pumped suction, the suction pressure should reach the red shade of the indicator scale and can be raised within 2 minutes.

Pull: The traction should be directed perpendicular to the cup. The left index and middle finger should be placed on the scalp. The thumb is placed on the anterior aspect of the cup while the right hand gives traction (Figure 15.1e). This step helps in detecting the descent of the fetus and warning us that the cup is getting detached. Lateral traction and rocking movement or rotational movement should be avoided at all costs. The line of the curve of Carus should be followed while giving traction. The station of the head, therefore, will guide the direction of traction. Once the head has descended to the perineum, the direction is changed to forward. The left hand moves to the posterior aspect of the cup and the scalp to prevent detachment. The traction is applied along with contraction and maternal pushing efforts. Episiotomy should be made if the perineum is stretching and threatening to tear.

The perineal support (Figure 15.1f): The attempt should be to bring (bunch up) the tissue of the perineum closer to the midline while supporting to prevent tear due to stretch. The delivery of the head at the perineum should be extremely slow. The mucocutaneous junction is slowly slipped off the head and the face of the fetus.

After delivery, one must explore the genital tract, including the cervix, for any tears.

When to abandon: Each traction should succeed in descending the fetus. With three pulls, usually, the head should be at the perineum and imminent to be born.

If two tractions did not succeed in any descent or if three pulls could not deliver the head or detachment of the cup more than once, then the procedure should be abandoned.

Rescue plan: When the vacuum fails, the options are to terminate by caesarean section or applying sequential forceps. The decision depends on the station and rotation of the head. Sequential instruments are reported to have a higher risk of adverse perinatal outcome and maternal soft tissue injuries. Therefore, it should be ventured into by experienced and skilled personnel only after taking the woman into confidence. In such a situation, one should be vigilant for post-delivery complications like shoulder dystocia and maternal complications like traumatic and atonic bleeding.

COMPLICATIONS

The complications of the extraction can be maternal or fetal.

MATERNAL COMPLICATIONS

These include

1. Bucket handle tear or annular avulsion of the cervix.
2. Vaginal bruising and tears or lacerations.
3. Post-partum haemorrhage due to trauma and atonicity due to prolonged labour, both are possible.
4. A complete perineal tear is likely if the position was wrongly assessed and the traction delivered a larger diameter or if the baby was big.

FETAL COMPLICATIONS

The most typical likely complication is cephalhematoma. There can be subgaleal haematoma which can sometimes expand and cause shock, severe anaemia, and later hyperbilirubinaemia in the newborn. There can be scalp avulsion or spiral tears on the fetal scalp that can happen if rotational traction is applied during traction in a malrotated head. Rarely there can be retinal haemorrhage and lateral rectus muscle injury to the fetus.

Prolonged labour and difficult vacuum-assisted delivery can result in birth asphyxia, hypoxic-ischaemic encephalopathy, and sepsis. There can be intracranial haemorrhage. Rarely, there can be neonatal death due to the impact of these morbidities.

Cephalhaematoma

This is blood collection under the periosteum of the skull (Figure 10.1c). Therefore, it is limited by sutures. It may not be present at birth and might take a few hours to manifest, and might gradually increase in size. This is an important differentiating feature from caput, which is always present at birth and progressively undergoes a reduction in size and resolution. Cephalhaematoma occurs due to trauma to the delicate vessels of the outer layer of the skull and the inner layer of the scalp. It is usually not associated with bleed inside the brain and is not likely to damage the brain. However, it may result in the development of hyperbilirubinaemia as it undergoes resolution by absorption. Rarely it can also cause anaemia if it is significant. The haematoma may resolve by absorption leaving behind a central soft crater-like area that can be indented in the middle with a hardness of calcification in the peripheries. It can happen spontaneously or due to the trauma of prolonged labour, cephalopelvic disproportion, and assisted vaginal birth with forceps or ventouse.

Subgaleal Hematoma

It is a bleed under the galeal aponeurosis but above the periosteum of the skull. So this is likely to cross the sutures and can spread to a large area on the skull. It is felt as a fluctuant mass. It might be present at birth and may expand later. It is due to bleeding from the vessels connecting the scalp vein to the dural sinuses. It is more life-threatening than cephalhematoma because it can become massive and is more likely to be associated with intracranial haemorrhage, skull fractures, and brain damage. It can cause shock (tachycardia pallor and low BP at birth or after that). It is likely to be due to the trauma of assisted delivery with forceps or ventouse, more often with latter. Imaging and specific treatment are needed to diagnose and manage associated cranial and brain injuries. Prematurity and underlying bleeding disorders can also be attributable to aetiology.

Subgaleal plane can lodge more than one-third of the baby's blood volume. Therefore, extreme vigilance for shock and anaemia is needed. Supportive treatment with blood transfusion might be necessary. Phototherapy is required to reduce hyperbilirubinaemia while it undergoes resolution. It can cause mortality in a fifth of the cases and so early diagnosis and prompt appropriate treatment are necessary.

DIFFERENCE IN VACUUM AND FORCEPS-ASSISTED DELIVERIES

Vacuum assistance can be used even when the cervical rim is palpable. Vacuum can be used for malrotated head, including deep transverse arrest. However, it should be avoided in a face to pubes delivery. Vacuum may not correct the asynclitism. Vacuum should be avoided in preterm fetuses.

Forceps are preferred over vacuum in the presence of caput and malpresentation like face or breech presentation.

In vacuum-assisted delivery, traction is given during contractions along with maternal efforts. In forceps, on the other hand, maternal efforts are not needed. That is why ventouse is not recommended for prophylactic use in a woman who should not bear down in the second stage of labour due to medical conditions like eclampsia or heart disease.

Vacuum is considered safer than forceps if appropriately applied, placing the cup at the flexion point. The risk of maternal injury is lesser with a vacuum if soft tissue entrapment is prevented. Vacuum assistance can cause cephalhematoma and subgaleal bleed.

Thus, ventouse-assisted delivery in an appropriately selected case is an asset in achieving successful vaginal birth and is likely to be associated with favourable maternal and perinatal outcomes.

16 Caesarean Section

Gowri Dorairajan
Jawaharlal Institute of Postgraduate Medical
Education and Research (JIPMER)

Caesarean section is the delivery of the fetus after incising the uterus through an abdominal incision. The rate of caesarean section is variable. It depends on the proportion of high-risk pregnancies in the concerned facility.

It depends on the type of facility management and the country. It is highest in the private sector in India.

INDICATIONS

These are broadly classified as fetal or maternal.
Fetal indications: The list is exhaustive. To enumerate, a few are

  i. Fetal distress (pathological CTG and women remote from the second stage)
 ii. Malpresentations like transverse lie and breech
iii. Growth-restricted fetus with abnormal dopplers
 iv. Cord presentation or prolapse
  v. Vasa previa
 vi. Active vaginal herpetic lesions
vii. Abruptio placenta with an alive salvageable fetus and woman remote from delivery

Maternal indications: The absolute indications are few, but the relative indication list is extensive. Following are the common indications:

a. Contracted pelvis.
b. Placenta previa.
c. Previous classical caesarean section/multiple lower segment scars/not eligible for a trial of labour after caesarean (TOLAC)/previous surgery involving the entire thickness of the upper segment like myomectomy.
d. Women who have undergone vesico-vaginal or high recto-vaginal fistula repairs.

There are many relative indications that are subject to variation, discussion, and sometimes criticism within the obstetric fraternity itself. A few of these are

1. **Precious pregnancy**: All pregnancies are precious to the concerned woman, but sometimes conception in older women following artificial techniques (in vitro fertilisation/ intracytoplasmic sperm injection/ donor semen or ovum), previous multiple abortions, and adverse perinatal outcome add to the preciousness and may compel a caesarean section.
2. **Previous caesarean section**: From simple refusal by the women, ineligibility, to lack of infrastructure for TOLAC can be taken as reasons for repeat scheduled caesarean sections.
3. Diabetic ketoacidosis.
4. PROM with failed induction.

DOI: 10.1201/9781003034360-16

5. Frank chorioamnionitis.
6. Impending renal shutdown in a woman with abruption. It is a rare indication and might have to be exercised even in the presence of intrauterine demise when the woman fails to respond to induction.

The list is exhaustive, as I earlier said.

Types of caesarean section
1. The caesarean section can be planned, scheduled (elective or pre-labour), or emergency.
2. Lower/upper segment (classical).
3. Transperitoneal/extraperitoneal.

Classical caesarean section is an incision placed in the upper segment of the uterus. The incision is a midline vertical incision in the upper segment of the uterus. It is indicated in the following few situations.

a. Placenta previa accrete or increta or percreta.
b. Woman with active cancer cervix.
c. In rare situations of extreme prematurity with placenta previa and malpresentation, a vertical incision may be necessary for the uterus to deliver the fetus.
d. Non-approachability to the lower segment, either due to dense adhesions of previous surgeries or due to large tumour-like fibroid occupying and distorting the lower segment, which is a rare instance.

In modern-day obstetrics, the caesarean section should be intended and completed as an intraperitoneal lower segment caesarean section. Extraperitoneal caesarean section was encouraged in cases of frank chorioamnionitis to avoid spillage of the infected liquor inside the peritoneal cavity. This technique requires exposing the lower segment by working in the pre-vesical extraperitoneal space. With the advent of antibiotics and advanced management facilities for infected cases, extraperitoneal caesarean section is a forgotten skill.

The classification for caesarean section can be based on urgency. In this regard, there are four categories (as laid down by NICE guidelines) [1].

I. Immediate threat to the life of woman or fetus: this is considered as "no delay" caesarean.
II. When there is a maternal and fetal compromise but not immediately life-threatening.
III. Requires early delivery. There is no maternal or fetal compromise.
IV. Delivery at a time suitable to the woman and the operating team.

One needs to audit and reduce the primary caesarean rate to as low as possible, balancing with the maternal and perinatal morbidity and mortality. In this regard, Robson had proposed a ten-group classification system referred to as TGCS or Robson's classification [2].

The WHO [3] endorsed the classification in 2015 to audit and monitor the indications in hospital facilities and recommends rates of around 10% at the population level. Caesarean section on demand is fortunately low in most parts of India.

PREOPERATIVE PREPARATIONS

Caesarean section is a major operation. Preoperative preparedness will reduce a few complications. Besides the **counselling and the consent**, a quick check on medical problems such as anaemia, abnormal blood sugars, and hypertension is essential. The elective caesarean section gives an ideal opportunity for overnight preparation. Blood should be crossmatched and available.

Caesarean cases should be preferably posted as the first case for operation. Any concurrent procedure like tubal ligation needs to be discussed with the woman and her partner. After counselling, written informed consent needs to be obtained.

Fasting: It is recommended that the woman should not take anything solid for 6–8 hours (or overnight fasting) and she should not take clear liquids at least 2 hours before the operation. Injection of H2 antagonists like ranitidine and metoclopramide will further reduce the risk of Mendelson syndrome [4]. An enema to empty the rectum has been considered to keep the woman comfortable in the postoperative period. However, this may not be possible for all women, especially when the caesarean is urgent, NICE I or II category. Recent trials have concluded that preoperative enema does not enhance postoperative bowel recovery or prevent gastrointestinal complications [5].

Hair removal: Most of the guidelines strongly recommend that shaving should be avoided. The hair should be removed with clippers if it is necessary [6].

Surgical antibiotic prophylaxis: Antibiotic prophylaxis is recommended by the ACOG [7] and must be followed within 60 minutes of the surgery. First-generation cephalosporins are the ones recommended (1–2 g of cefazolin depending on the weight of the woman).

Urinary self-retaining Foley catheter is inserted immediately before the operation to ensure the urinary bladder is kept empty.

Choice anaesthesia: Regional anaesthesia through the subarachnoid block (spinal) is the preferred anaesthesia for most caesarean sections. It ensures anaesthesia and motor block without hindering the uterine contractions. In addition, one should place a lateral wedge under the woman's back to prevent hypotension in the supine position.

In certain situations like severe fetal bradycardia and cord prolapse, we may have to insist on general anaesthesia. It is prudent to do caesareans for placenta previa and placenta accreta under general anaesthesia for reasonable control of respiration and circulation as these cases are likely to be associated with sudden severe life-threatening blood loss. In placental adhesive disorders, such as accreta and increta, it is mandatory to operate under general anaesthesia. If need be, arterial lines can be placed before proceeding with the surgery to monitor arterial pressure.

SKIN INCISION AND STEPS

The skin and abdominal wall can be incised by either a midline sub-umbilical vertical incision or horizontal suprapubic transverse incision.

Vertical incision: Sub-umbilical midline vertical incision is the most avascular and gives the fastest entry into the abdominal cavity. Every obstetrician should be well versed with this incision. The author prefers this incision over a suprapubic transverse incision in the following situations:

Second stage caesareans, placenta previa, or accreta, when there is a concurrent problem like an ovarian cyst and certain situations of acute fetal bradycardia associated with abruption or cord prolapse. The vertical abdominal incision is also preferred whenever a classical caesarean section is contemplated or becomes necessary.

Disadvantages of vertical incision are more pain, more strain on the wound, and chances of hernia formation, and it is considered cosmetically inferior.

Pfannenstiel incision (Kerr incision): Opening of the abdomen by low transverse suprapubic incision. The incision is kept just above the pubic symphysis, so the hairline will later almost cover the incision. A horizontal incision that is slightly curved at the ends is made on the skin and deepened to the subcutaneous fat till the rectus sheath. The rectus sheath is cut horizontally to get access to the abdominal cavity. The rectus muscles are separated along the midline raphe and retracted laterally. The posterior rectus sheath above the arcuate line and the fascia transversalis below is incised, and the peritoneum is opened vertically. One must be careful while retracting the muscles laterally. There is a risk of injuring the vessels under the muscle, and life-threatening hematomas can form under the rectus sheath. For this reason, the author avoids this incision in patients who have preoperative coagulation failures like severe abruption or liver failure cases.

In the incision described by Rapin and Kustner, the rectus sheath was incised vertically.

The *advantage* of Pfannenstiel's incision is that it is cosmetically better. It has better healing as it is along the lines of anterior abdominal wall expression. The tension along the rectus sheath in transverse incision is much less than that in vertical incisions, and so, there is a lesser risk of herniation through it. It is associated with less pain in the postoperative period.

Disadvantages: The scar becomes uncomfortable when the pubic hair grows back. The formation of panniculus increases the humidity and warmth around the scar area, increasing the risk of infection in obese women. A higher incision called the Joel-Cohen incision does not have these disadvantages. It was introduced by Professor Joel-Cohen in 1974. The skin is incised 3 cm below the line joining the anterior superior iliac spines. The subcutaneous tissue and the rectus sheath are incised horizontally only in the midline. Thereafter the tissue, including fat and rectus sheath, is split open by finger dissection. Splitting avoids cutting a lot of vessels, including perforator vessels. The rectus muscle is retracted laterally. The parietal peritoneum is opened at a point as high as possible and incised vertically downwards. It is a good idea to incise the peritoneal under vision by sharp dissection rather than bluntly by finger dissection. Picking up the peritoneum between two artery forceps and ensuring translucency or palpating to rule out any intraperitoneal contents before incising is an important step to prevent accidental injury to the abdominal viscera like intestine.

Steps of Caesarean Section

After opening the abdomen by any of these methods, one enters the abdominal cavity. It is important now to expose the lower part of the uterus and *visualise the two round ligaments*. This step will prevent accidental incisions on the lateral or the posterior surface of the uterus. There have been instances where the posterior wall of the lower segment was incised because the uterus was 360° rotated. Visualising the lower segment and *correcting any version* would ensure that the incision is on the anterior wall of the lower segment. If one of the round ligaments is anterior, it means that the uterus is verted. The version can be corrected by rotating the uterus back to normal and putting a mop pack behind the opposite round ligament. The mop will prevent the rotated uterus from falling back to where it was. If the version is not corrected, then the incision is likely to open into engorged vessels and extend to involve the uterine artery causing brisk haemorrhage.

Identify the *loose utero-vesical fold of the peritoneum*. The lower segment lies below this loose fold of the peritoneum. The utero-vesical fold of the peritoneum should be incised with scissors, and the bladder is pushed down with blunt dissection and retracted by the Doyens retractor to keep the bladder away from the operating field. In cases with previous caesarean section, blunt dissection should be avoided, and sharp dissection is preferred to release the adhesions to free the bladder. Thus, the *lower segment is identified* as the segment under the utero-vesical fold of the peritoneum and is situated below and between the two round ligaments. The lower segment is now incised in a curvilinear manner with scissors. The lower segment can also be opened by making an initial horizontal window in the midline and then with finger splitting to the sides by both the index fingers. The membranes can now be ruptured by twisting with artery forceps or nicking with the scissors. The fetus is delivered out. In vertex presentation, we should ensure that the flexion of the head is maintained so that the smallest diameter of the fetal head exits the incision. This step is important to prevent the extension of the lower segment incision. The *angles of the incision are held* with the Green Armitage forceps if there is a vessel spurting blood; otherwise, Allis tissue holding forceps can also be used. The angles can be secured with ligatures as one awaits placental separation. There is no need to do a manual removal of the placenta as a routine. It is essential to identify the lower flap of the lower segment and not mistake the protruding posterior wall of the lower segment to be the lower flap. One can confirm this by sliding the finger on the inner aspect of the held flap of the lower segment to reach the internal os. *The internal os can also be dilated* with a finger or with Hegar's dilator if the os was closed, as happens in pre-labour caesarean sections. *The uterus is closed in two layers*, excluding the decidual layer as continuous suturing. Locking sutures should be avoided as it compromises the blood supply. The *second layer should bury*

(Lambert) the first layer completely. It is best achieved if the first layer needle bites are taken as close to the edge of the incision as possible and taking the needle entry-exit site of the second layer well beyond the needle insertion site of the first layer (Figure 16.1a). This step will ensure proper railroad and will bury the first layer. As a practice, the author closes the visceral peritoneum also. The ovaries should always be visualised for any pathologies to do any concurrent surgery in the same sitting. If the woman had consented earlier, then tubectomy can be performed by modified Pomeroy's technique.

The peritoneal cavity is cleared of all the blood or amniotic fluid. Then instrument and mop count is checked before closing back the abdomen in layers. The parietal peritoneum need not be closed, and the rectus muscle needs to be only apposed in the midline. There is no need to approximate the rectus muscle with sutures as it is associated with increased postoperative pain. The rectus sheath should be sutured with delayed absorbable like polyglactin or non-absorbable suture-like polypropylene. Catgut should not be used for rectus sheath. The subcutaneous fat needs to be approximated with sutures if it is more than 2 cm deep. The skin can be closed with absorbable subcuticular sutures. In the original Joel-Cohen technique, the skin is closed by subcuticular sutures. In the original Misgav Ladach technique, the skin is closed with interrupted sutures. The choice rests on the individual surgeon and the circumstances and facility concerned.

VARIOUS TECHNIQUES [8]

Pfannenstiel technique: The skin incision is by Pfannenstiel incision as described above. The uterus is closed in two layers with continuous sutures and closure to the peritoneum's visceral and parietal layers.

In the *Joel-Cohen technique* of caesarean section, the uterus is closed in a single layer by interrupted stitches, and the visceral peritoneum is not closed.

In the *Misgav Ladach technique*, the abdomen is opened by the Joel-Cohen technique. The uterus is closed with a single layer of continuous sutures, and the peritoneum is not sutured.

Any combination of the above methods with Joel-Cohen technique for opening the abdomen and double-layer closure of the uterus is called as modified Misgav Ladach technique. In the meta-analysis comparing the Pfannenstiel and the Joel-Cohen-based approach, the latter was more effective and had more advantages and is, therefore, recommended [9].

The Coronis trial [10] was the largest trial to answer the controversies on abdominal entry by incision or blunt dissection technique, closure of the uterus by a double or single layer, closure or not of visceral peritoneum, and type of suture for uterine closure. The trial concluded that either method is acceptable. This trial studied only short-term outcomes. The follow-up trial [11] showed that there was no difference in the primary outcome in the aspects regarding the technique of entry into the abdomen, exteriorisation or not of the uterus while suturing, closure or not of visceral peritoneum, and polyglactin versus catgut use for suturing uterus. The follow-up study did not find any difference in the rate of rupture in subsequent pregnancy based on single- or double-layer closure of the uterus. However, the follow-up was not powered to detect serious adverse events. Only 20% of women in both groups had a subsequent pregnancy. I would recommend double-layer closure especially for women who are likely to have future pregnancies, as it does not significantly increase the operating time.

DIFFICULT CAESAREAN SECTION: HOW TO BAIL ONESELF OUT

It is vital to perform the caesarean section safely and swiftly. This will not only ensure maternal and perinatal safety but help gain the trust of the operating team, including the scrub nurse and the anaesthetist.

In caesareans where difficulties are anticipated, it is essential to plan well. Following are the situations where one must expect difficulties:

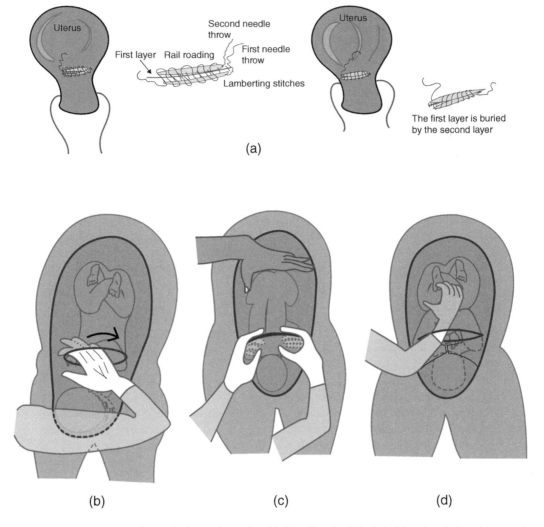

FIGURE 16.1 a) Lamberting technique of suturing. b) Anterior shoulder is held and pulled to the opposite side to make back anterior. c) Line diagram showing Patwardhan technique of fetal delivery. d) Reverse breech delivery technique.

   i. Pre-labour preterm (less than 32 weeks) caesareans section with malpresentation and decreased amniotic fluid due to rupture of membranes.
  ii. Free-floating head with placenta previa.
 iii. Caesarean section for placenta previa.
  iv. Caesarean for previous two or more caesarean scars.
   v. Second stage caesarean section.
  vi. Caesarean sections for adhesive placental disorders like placenta previa accreta or increta.
 vii. Caesareans performed for a transverse lie.

These situations can sometimes become highly demanding. Therefore, the obstetrician needs to anticipate problems and plan each step well.

Let us look at some details of the tricks for the above situations.

Preparedness: When difficulties are expected, it is a good idea to have reasonable assistance. Have a senior paediatrician available to resuscitate the baby. Keep blood arranged beforehand. The anaesthetists should be informed prior regarding possibilities of bleeding as a complication and the likely extended time of operation so that they can plan the anaesthesia accordingly. Before scrubbing up, one should know the exact position of the fetus and its back, especially so in transverse lie.

The other important planning is to arrange for a pair of obstetric forceps or Kiwi's vacuum cup in the caesarean trolley.

The choice of skin incision must be based on the likely difficulty in delivery, the BMI of the woman, previous surgeries, and the indication for the index caesarean section.

A vertical incision to open the abdominal wall should be preferred when a classical caesarean is proposed or when there are many previous suprapubic incisions and there is dense fibrosis expected. The author prefers vertical incision for caesareans in the second stage and obstructed labour.

Uterine incision: We should restrict the uterine incision to the lower segment only as far as possible. It may be tricky to deliver a fetus with malpresentation from a preterm tubular lower segment. A vertical incision on the lower segment is attended with the risk of extension to the upper segment above or the fornix below.

To increase the available incised space in a preterm caesarean, one should make a U-shaped incision in the lower segment. To achieve this, the bladder should be pushed as low down as possible. It can be done with finger dissection after opening the utero-vesical fold of the peritoneum or by sharp dissection. The horizontal limb of the U-shaped incision should be placed in the lowest part of the lower segment in the midline parallel to the lower segment. After that, it should be curved up on both sides as "U". This would tremendously increase the available space. While extracting as breech, one must remember the crucial goal of preventing head entrapment. At times of crisis, one may have to extend one of the "U" vertical limbs upwards like a "J". This will avoid accidental extension to involve the uterine arteries in the lateral aspect. The alternative is to give a vertical incision downwards, "T"- shaped incision, but this is fraught with the serious problem of extension to the fornix below.

Delivery of the fetus

A. **Caesarean section for vertex presentations**: In vertex presentation for a right-handed surgeon, the dominant right hand is placed in the cavity of the uterus through the incised lower uterine segment below the fetal head. The head is gently lifted out of the incision. The Doyens retractor is removed after getting a firm grip on the head before lifting it out of the incision. One must lift the head from occiput to sinciput direction to ensure the head remains flexed while delivering. Hence, the importance of knowing the position of the fetus before starting the caesarean section. The shoulders are delivered by gentle upward and downward traction.

B. **Free-floating head**: In such a situation, before starting a caesarean, the operator should be sure about the back position. The same principle as above is followed, but the non-dominant hand of the operator should steady the pole of the head just above the upper edge of the incision (from over the abdominal wall) with firm, steady pressure. This will prevent the free-floating head from escaping the higher cephalad or into the side of the uterine cavity. It will also help the dominant hand get a firm grip on the head. This is aided by the fundal pressure by the assistant to extract the free head.

Suppose this fails to deliver the head out, then as an alternative, one can use Wrigley's outlet forceps with cephalic application to grip and extract the head after locking the blades. Cephalic application of the forceps needs to be done to extract a free head.

The other way is to use the Kiwi's vacuum pump. The application should be close to the occiput in the midline (flexion point) of the head to prevent deflexion while delivering.

Suppose none of the above manoeuvres work and obstetric forceps or vacuum is not readily available and the timing is running out after uterine incision. In that case, one should insert the dominant hand right inside the uterine fundus to hold the feet and extract the fetus as a breech.

C. **Caesarean for transverse lie**: One should know the exact position of the back, head, and limbs. This is important as it would guide the obstetrician as to which part of the fundus to approach to hold the feet of the fetus and deliver out the baby by breech extraction. If time is wasted in discovering the fetal parts after the uterine incision is made, then the liquor might flow out and make the delivery more and more difficult. One may end up holding the hand and bringing it out of the incision. Delivering the hand would create a problem by reducing the available space and wasting time in repositing the hand and feeling for the feet. This is particularly difficult in situations where liquor has already got drained or placenta previa as every second after incising uterus or cutting through the placenta matters for neonatal survival. The uterine incision should be adequate (as described in the above section) to prevent head entrapment.

D. **Caesarean for placenta previa**: Before proceeding with the caesarean, one should know the position and type of placenta previa. The maximum problem for fetal delivery occurs in type II or III anterior placenta previa. The placenta is likely to be cut as it comes under the incision on the lower segment. The fetus can, therefore, get exsanguinated. Cutting through the placenta is a serious risk of exsanguination of the fetus and demands brisk delivery of the fetus. If the placenta is type III or IV anterior, then one should make the incision on the lower segment as high as possible to be able to approach the membranes at the upper edge of the placenta. This way will avoid cutting through the placenta. If the placenta is anterior type II, the surgeon should place the incision on the lower segment as low as possible to approach the membrane through the lower edge of the placenta. This can help to avoid cutting through the placenta. After incising the lower segment, one should approach the membrane and do an amniotomy to reach the fetus. If, however, it is not possible to reach any of the edges of the placenta, then one has to cut through the placenta. In such a situation, one must be extremely swift in delivering the fetus and has to be precise in identifying the fetal feet to deliver as breech or grip the high head firmly and deliver. There is no scope or opportunity to use a vacuum or forceps to deliver the head as the pool of blood in the field will make the visualisation and the application difficult. Also, there is a serious risk of exsanguination and asphyxia if the delivery of the fetus after cutting the placenta is delayed.

E. **Caesarean section in the second stage**

It is vital to plan these caesareans properly. There can be difficulties in various steps.

i. *Catheterisation of the urinary bladder* may be difficult because the urethrovesical junction may be kinked or compressed due to the jammed head. Therefore, inserting the palmar aspect of the non-dominant head in the vagina to elevate the urethrovesical junction to align the urethra and bladder in line may be necessary to aid in catheter insertion.

ii. *Planning the incision* in caesarean section can be accomplished with the Joel-Cohen technique with the suprapubic transverse incision. A vertical incision might be useful when the bladder appears oedematous, stretched, and advanced, and there is obstructed labour.

iii. *The parietal peritoneum needs to be opened as high as possible* in a transparent area. The bladder might be stretched, oedematous, and pulled up and advanced up to the umbilicus sometimes. One might inadvertently incise the urinary bladder if this precaution is not followed.

iv. The lower segment might be stretched and sometimes extremely thinned or ballooned out in the presence of obstructed labour. The incision on the *lower segment should **not** be very low* as it may be opening into the anterior vagina (laproelytrotomy) [12,13]. The incision on the lower segment should therefore be kept reasonably high in the stretched lower segment.

Delivery of the fetus in second stage caesarean section: When the fetal head is impacted in the pelvis, there can be problems in delivering the head, and one needs to plan the steps. One should be aware of the vaginal examination findings, position, and the station of the head. The decision of the method to deliver the fetus also depends on what part presents at the uterine incision.

DELIVERY AS HEAD

If the ears or the fetus's neck shows up at the uterine incision, the attempt should be to deliver it as the head. For this, the dominant hand should slide deep into the pelvis over and then beyond and below the head. Slight lifting will undo the suction in the pelvis and release the impacted head. The head can then be delivered, upholding the principle of keeping the head flexed.

PUSH METHOD

Vaginal assistance to push the head up is an alternative if the neck presents at the uterine incision and the head is deep in the pelvis. An assistant should introduce a gloved hand in the vagina and push the head up with a cupped hand with even pressure on the head, maintaining flexion (force from occiput towards sinciput). Thus the head is lifted, and the suction is released. The operator from above can get a firm grip by placing the dominant hand well below the head and deliver the head from the incision as the vertex. One blade of the forceps can be used as a Vectis. It should be introduced along with the head under cover of the hand, protecting the lower segment flap. The forceps blade is introduced to the posterior parietal bone, and the head is lifted with the forceps blade to undo the suction created in the pelvis. Thereafter, the fetus can be delivered as the vertex.

THE SHOULDER PRESENTS AT THE UTERINE INCISION

a. Patwardhan technique: This is necessary when the shoulders are present at the uterine incision. Keeping the incision deliberatively high in the lower segment will ensure that the shoulders present at the incision. The fetus can be delivered by the following methods (Figure 16.1b and c). The anterior shoulder is pulled to the one side to bring the back anterior and bring the opposite shoulder also at the incision site. The index and middle fingers are introduced along the chest wall side, and the trunk is flexed. This aided by fundal pressure from assistant delivers the chest, abdomen, and buttocks, and then the breech is delivered in that order. This is followed by delivery of the head. The fetus somersaults and delivers out. This is a safe method of delivery. This was described way back in 1957.

b. In the second method, the anterior shoulder is delivered first. One hand of the operator inserted along the ventrum of the fetus holds the foot of the anterior leg, and the same is delivered out. This is followed by delivery of the other leg and buttocks in that order. The back is kept anterior. Traction is given to deliver the other shoulder and arm. The head follows last.

c. Pull method or reverse breech method for the occipito-transverse position. In occipito transverse or posterior position, when one shoulder presents at the uterine incision, then the operator's hand is inserted in the fundus of the uterus to grasp the foot of the anterior leg. With traction, the anterior leg followed by the posterior leg and then the buttocks are delivered in that order. Thereafter, the trunk is delivered, and the fundus is emptied, and the shoulders and the head get automatically disengaged with the traction on the buttocks and trunk. The shoulders and the head are sequentially delivered out.

If on incising the lower segment, the chest and nipples of the baby present (direct occipito posterior position (Figure 16.1d)). In such a situation, the operator's dominant hand should be introduced along the ventral aspect of the chest and abdomen to hold the feet. The buttocks, trunk, and shoulders follow the two legs and lastly, the head is delivered out.

FETAL PILLOW DEVICE

This has been tested and found to aid in faster delivery. The device is inserted from below on the fetal head and inflated to push up the head from the pelvis [14].

The Patwardhan and the reverse breech technique were found to be safer than the push method in terms of lower segment extensions of the incision line, amount of blood loss, and infection rates [15–17].

TROUBLED SITUATIONS

EXTENSION OF THE INCISION

Extension of the incision made on the lower segment is likely to occur in difficult caesarean sections. It happens more often in the second stage caesareans for obstructed labour and deeply engaged head. It can also occur spontaneously or extended deliberately by the operator due to the panic experienced while delivering a fetus with malpresentation, especially when also preterm.

The extension can occur towards the lateral side and may open into the uterine artery or venous plexus or extend vertically downwards in the lower segment. Sometimes the vertical extensions may involve the anterior vagina down to the bladder base.

We need to prevent extensions by planning and executing the caesarean section as described in this chapter already.

Lateral extension: The extension may go upwards towards the upper segment or to the side to involve the uterine arteries or sometimes even the posterior aspect of the lower segment. It is essential to recognise that it has occurred. So, suppose the intact edge beyond the apex is not visualised, then one can even exteriorise the uterus to observe and define the limits of the incision and recognise the extension. In the absence of bleeding for the uterine artery, one can start suturing from beyond the apex of the new angle. The palmar surface of the non-dominant hand of the operator should lift the posterior aspect of the broad ligament and guide the suturing of the lateral extension so that the suture does not inadvertently go through the posterior leaf of the broad ligament, in the event of which hematoma can form from the venous plexus in the broad ligament as well as from the infundibulopelvic vessels. The finger guard will also prevent inadvertent deep posterior suture

---

TABLE 16.1

Showing the Delivery Technique at the Caesarean Section for Second Stage Deeply Engaged Head

Order of the Fetal Part Delivered	Patwardhan OT Position Deeply Engaged Anterior Shoulder Presenting at the Incision	Reverse Breech1 OP/OT Deeply Engaged Head, Anterior Shoulder Presenting at the Incision	Reverse Breech2 (Deeply Engaged DOP Front of Chest Presenting)
1	Anterior shoulder	Anterior shoulder	Anterior leg
2	Posterior shoulder	Anterior leg	Posterior leg
3	Trunk	Posterior leg	Buttocks
4	Buttocks	buttocks	trunk
5	One leg	Trunk	One shoulder
6	Another leg	Posterior shoulder	Second shoulder
7	Face then vertex	Vertex then face	Vertex then face

bites that can kink or involve the ureters. The lateral extension can be sutured with a single layer by continuous or interrupted sutures.

Vertical extension: Vertical downward extension on the lower segment can be tricky because sometimes they may extend to the anterior vagina. This is more likely to happen in caesareans done at full dilation. These vertical downward extensions can be sutured with continuous or interrupted single or double layer depending on the friability and thickness of the edges. Sometimes double layering can cause button-hole tears if the tissues are very thinned out. The idea is to ensure haemostasis and achieve closure. Non-braided suture-like catgut may be a better option while suturing thinned out friable lower segment. The bladder may have to be pushed down further to visualise beyond the lower apex of the extension. It should be sutured separately from the main incision to restore the anatomy of the lower flap, to secure haemostasis, and ensure complete approximation. The non-dominant hand inserted from within the lower flap of the lower segment will help visualise the extension's margins.

The J-shaped extension in the upper segment should be sutured in one layer to ensure approximation and haemostasis. It may not be possible to achieve double-layer closure.

Broad ligament hematoma: During a difficult delivery of the impacted presenting part, the extension of the uterine incision may open into the uterine vessel resulting in the formation of hematoma in between the two leaves of the broad ligament.

It is a good practice opening the anterior leaf of the broad ligament when a hematoma has formed. The next step could be to evacuate the hematoma and identify the bleeder. It may become extremely challenging to locate the bleeder because of the brisk pool of blood that forms on evacuating the hematoma, and the vessel retracts laterally. The bleeding vessel should preferably be identified and ligated. Blind haemostatic suture bites in the retroperitoneal space are extremely risky and are the most typical reason for postoperative uretero-vaginal fistula formation or ipsilateral ureteric ligation or partial injury of the ureter.

The second approach is to ligate the anterior division of the hypogastric artery of the same side first and then empty the hematoma, especially when the hematoma is large. Sometimes it may be necessary to ligate the uterine artery at its origin from the internal iliac artery. Uterine vein injury has to be dealt with similarly by identifying the venous plexus and ligating them carefully proximally. Tamponade with surgical mops left for 24–48 hours is the last resort. It is not followed anymore as this procedure needs a relaparotomy to remove the mops. Also, as the bleeding is traumatic, it is amenable to primary haemostatic suturing. The operating surgeon must be well versed with uterine artery and internal iliac artery ligation or should take prompt help from those with expertise when needed. It is a good dictum to delineate the course of the ureter once the bleeding has been controlled to rule out any ureteric injury/ligation. A cystoscopy can also be done to look at the free intravesical spurting of urine from both ureters.

Embolising the uterine artery may not be readily available in all setups and is not feasible in an unanticipated emergency. One can place a catheter in the internal iliac artery retrograde from the femoral artery before performing a planned caesarean section. The embolisation can be done after delivering the baby by caesarean section.

ELYTROTOMY

It is a condition where the incision on the lower segment during a caesarean section has been inadvertently placed in the anterior vaginal wall. This situation can be encountered when the caesarean section is being done for obstructed labour or late in the second stage. It is imperative to recognise this and suture the rent in the anterior vaginal wall [12]. One can re-suture the anterior vagina wall to the avulsed cervix [13]. It becomes challenging to identify this condition when the caesarean section is being done in the second stage of labour because the cervix cannot be identified easily and separately from the vagina.

I want to **narrate a case**. I was called by the registrar on duty to the operation theatre after he had delivered the fetus. The caesarean section was being done for second stage arrest in a second gravida. After delivery of the fetus, the registrar could not establish the anatomy of the incised part, and there was brisk bleeding. When I examined, the upper flap of the uterus appeared to be completely detached all around circularly. The cervix or the lower flap was not identifiable. I had to do an intra-operator vaginal examination to understand the anatomy. I could see the gloved finger inserted in the vagina in the abdominal field. The utero-cervix appeared to have got wholly detached all around from the vagina. Since the cervix was not specifically identifiable, I had to resort to a hysterectomy and closure of the vagina. In this case, the elytrotomy had possibly extended all around and detached the vagina from the utero-cervix around all fornices. Therefore, it is prudent to keep the incision higher (only about one or two centimetres below the utero-vesical peritoneal fold) to prevent accidental vaginal incision and delivery of the fetus from the vagina when the lower segment appears to be extremely stretched out.

POSTOPERATIVE CARE

Postoperative care depends on the indication of the caesarean section and whether it was planned scheduled or an emergency in labour. If a planned, scheduled caesarean is performed in a primigravida, postoperative care should be towards early recovery after surgery (ERAS).

Postoperative pain relief is essential for the early ambulation of a woman. Most of the caesarean sections are performed under regional or neuro-axial anaesthesia.

One should add parenteral analgesia with an opioid, for example, morphine or fentanyl, to relieve pain in the postoperative period. At the same time, the use of parenteral analgesics should be kept to minimal as she must be wakeful to feed and nurse the neonate. One can use nonsteroidal anti-inflammatory drugs like diclofenac or ketorolac, or paracetamol. The choice of the drug depends on the patient preference, allergies, and side effects. Transversus abdominis plane block is found to give substantial pain relief.

Intravenous fluids and nutrition: The fluid requirement varies depending on how long before the caesarean she was fasting. The requirement goes up tremendously in women undergoing caesarean late in labour when the caesarean lasts longer than 1 hour, and there was extensive dissection due to adhesions. The women who are taken for caesarean in the second stage of labour and were dehydrated even before the delivery also require more intravenous fluids. The need also goes up when there is a rise in temperature. The requirement could therefore vary from 100 mL/hour to up to 200 mL/hour. The fluids are usually ringer lactate and 5% dextrose drip. A saline infusion may be needed when there was baseline dehydration and exhaustion during labour. The urine output should be at least 50 mL/hour. After most of the routine caesarean sections, early feeding can be resumed within 6 hours of delivery. The exceptions are women who had bowel distension due to obstructed labour or those where extensive bowel and omental adhesions were dissected.

Antibiotics: Usually, prophylactic antibiotics are sufficient. The antibiotics are extended as therapeutic in caesareans done for chorioamnionitis/prolonged second stage/extensive adhesion dissection/placenta previa cases or as per the individual case. The antibiotic policy of the respective centre should be followed.

Thromboprophylaxis: This may be needed in some cases. The Royal College (RCOG) has laid the criteria for the same. Enoxaparin or heparin can be started 6–12 hours after surgery.

The urinary bladder catheter can be removed in 12–24 hours. Prolonged catheterisation for 3–5 days is recommended in women with oedematous and stretched-out urinary bladder. The woman who underwent caesarean section for obstructed labour needs to have bladder rest for 7 days to prevent the formation of an obstetric vesical-vaginal fistula.

The woman should be mobilised as early as possible (at least within 8–10 hours of surgery).

The woman can be allowed to bathe the next day. The sutures are usually removed after 7 days. However, most of the centres are now using absorbable subcuticular sutures.

Early recovery after surgery protocols for caesarean section varies between centres and countries [18]. The components consistently included are early initiation of oral feed, early ambulation, and early removal of the catheter. The ERAS protocols have shown to be very useful in shortening hospital stays and hastening recovery [19,20].

REFERENCES

1. Classification of Urgency of Caesarean Section – RCOG. https://www.rcog.org.uk > documents > guidelines. No. 11-Apr-2010.
2. Robson, MS. Classification of caesarean sections. *Fetal Matern Med Rev.* 2001;12(1):23–39.
3. World Health Organization. *WHO Statement on Caesarean Section Rates.* Geneva: World Health Organization; 2015. (WHO/RHR/15.02).
4. American Society of Anesthesiologists Task Force on Obstetric Anesthesia. Practice guidelines for obstetric anesthesia: An updated report by the American society of anesthesiologists task force on obstetric anesthesia. *Anesthesiology.* 2016;124(2):270–300.
5. Ertas IE, Ince O, Emirdar V, Gultekin E, Biler A, Kurt S. Influence of preoperative enema application on the return of gastrointestinal function in elective Cesarean sections: a randomised controlled trial. *J Matern Fetal Neonatal Med.* 2021;34(11):1822–1826. doi: 10.1080/14767058.2019.1651264. Epub 2019 Aug 9. PMID: 31397204.
6. ACOG Practice Bulletin No. 199 Summary: Use of Prophylactic Antibiotics in Labor and Delivery. *Obstet Gynecol.* 2018;132(3):798–800. doi: 10.1097/AOG.0000000000002834.
7. Allegranzi B, Bischoff P, de Jonge S, Kubilay N, Zayed B, Gomes S, Abbas M, Atema J, Gans S, Rijen M, Boermeester M, Egger M, Kluytmans J, Pittet D, Solomkin J. New WHO recommendations on preoperative measures for surgical site infection prevention: an evidence-based global perspective. *Lancet Infect Dis.* 2016;16. doi: 10.1016/S1473-3099(16)30398-X.
8. Hofmeyr GJ, Mathai M, Shah AN, Novikova N. Techniques for caesarean section. *Cochr Lib.* 2008;(1):CD004662. doi: 10.1002/14651858.CD004662.pub2. PMID: 18254057.
9. Olyaeemanesh A, Bavandpour E, Mobinizadeh M, Ashrafinia M, Bavandpour M, Nouhi M. Comparison of the Joel-Cohen-based technique and the transverse Pfannenstiel for caesarean section for safety and effectiveness: A systematic review and meta analysis. *Med J Islam Repub Iran.* 2017;31:54. doi: 10.14196/mjiri.31.54.
10. CORONIS Collaborative Group, Abalos E, Addo V, Brocklehurst P, El Sheikh M, Farrell B, Gray S, Hardy P, Juszczak E, Mathews JE, Masood SN, Oyarzun E, Oyieke J, Sharma JB, Spark P. Caesarean section surgical techniques (CORONIS): A fractional, factorial, unmasked, randomised controlled trial. *Lancet.* 2013;382(9888):234–248. doi: 10.1016/S0140-6736(13)60441-9. Epub 2013 May 28.
11. CORONIS collaborative group, Abalos E, Addo V, Brocklehurst P, El Sheikh M, Farrell B, Gray S, Hardy P, Juszczak E, Mathews JE, Naz Masood S, Oyarzun E, Oyieke J, Sharma JB, Spark P. Caesarean section surgical techniques: 3-year follow-up of the CORONIS fractional, factorial, unmasked, randomised controlled trial The CORONIS collaborative group. *Lancet.* 2016;388(10039):62–72. doi: 10.1016/S0140-6736(16)00204-X.
12. Rashid M. Accidental delivery of a baby during a caesarean section through a vaginal incision (a laparoelytrotomy). *BMJ Case Rep.* 2010;2010:bcr0720103135. doi: 10.1136/bcr.07.2010.3135.
13. Gortzak-Uzan L, Walfisch A, Gortzak Y, Katz M, Mazor M, Hallak M. Accidental vaginal incision during cesarean section. A report of four cases. *J Reprod Med.* 2001;46(11):1017–20
14. Lassey SC, Little SE, Saadeh M, et al. Cephalic elevation device for second-stage cesarean delivery: A randomized controlled trial. *Obstet Gynecol.* 2020;135(4):879–884. doi: 10.1097/AOG.0000000000003746.
15. Lenz, F., Kimmich, N., Zimmermann, R. *et al.* Maternal and neonatal outcome of reverse breech extraction of an impacted fetal head during caesarean section in advanced stage of labour: a retrospective cohort study. *BMC Pregnancy Childbirth* 2019;19, 98. doi: 10.1186/s12884-019-2253-3.
16. Jeve YB, Navti OB, Konje JC. Comparison of techniques used to deliver a deeply impacted fetal head at full dilation: a systematic review and meta-analysis. *BJOG.* 2016;123(3):337–345. doi: 10.1111/1471-0528.13593.

17. Berhan Y, Berhan A. A meta-analysis of reverse breech extraction to deliver a deeply impacted head during cesarean delivery. *Int J Gynaecol Obstet.* 2014;124(2):99–105. Epub 2013 Nov 6.

18. Ituk U, Habib AS. Enhanced recovery after cesarean delivery. *F1000Res.* 2018;7:F1000 Faculty Rev-513. doi: 10.12688/f1000research.13895.1.

19. Sajidah Ilyas, Scott Simmons, Sohail Bampoe. Systematic review of enhanced recovery protocols for elective caesarean section versus conventional care. *Aust N Z J Obstet Gynaecol.* 2019;59(6):767–776.

20. Corso, E., Hind, D., Beever, D. *et al.* Enhanced recovery after elective caesarean: a rapid review of clinical protocols, and an umbrella review of systematic reviews. *BMC Pregnancy Childbirth* 2017;17:91. doi: 10.1186/s12884-017-1265-0.

17 Post-Partum Haemorrhage

Gowri Dorairajan
Jawaharlal Institute of Postgraduate Medical
Education and Research (JIPMER)

Post-partum haemorrhage (PPH) remains a significant cause of maternal mortality, especially in developing countries. No woman should die of a post-partum haemorrhage. Anticipation through risk assessment and universal prevention by active management are essential strategies towards reducing post-partum haemorrhage. Blood loss is always underestimated. Early detection, prompt resuscitation, and definitive management are essential strategies to avert maternal death. This chapter deals with the definition as well as the risk factors of PPH. This chapter details the objective definition. The chapter also sensitizes the caregiving team to identify excess bleed and flag a case as likely excessive bleeding so that the team gets alerted for further preparedness and action.

DEFINITION

There are various definitions of post-partum haemorrhage.

Traditionally, it is defined as blood loss above 500 mL after vaginal delivery and more than 1,000 mL after caesarean delivery (RCOG) [1]. Objective quantification of blood loss is difficult at birth. There is always an underestimation of blood loss. So, the other definition (ACOG) [2] refers to any amount of bleeding from or into the genital tract that makes the patient symptomatic (light headache, vertigo, syncope, tachycardia, hypotension, and oliguria). The bleeding can immediately follow the birth of a baby or can occur anytime till the end of puerperium. It is also defined as any bleeding that decreases haematocrit by 10% or requiring blood transfusion.

CLINICAL IDENTIFICATION

Visual estimation of blood loss is always underestimated and may not be objectively measurable at each delivery due to logistic constraints. Objective measurement with blood collection bag drapes will give better estimates but may not always be feasible or accurate, especially with amniotic fluid contamination. The blood collection devices may not always be available in all set-ups. Pictorial guidelines might give quick alerts and assessments of blood loss. Given that the first hour is the golden hour in managing PPH and preventing its complications, it is essential to recognize it as early as possible. In high turnover labour rooms of big government and or teaching hospitals, the labour or delivery might be attended by nursing students as well as medical students under training. In the interest of good outcome, in high turnover centres with heterogenous qualification of the caregivers, it is prudent to get alerted and inform the next senior in the team as soon as one sees a clot at the time of delivery or a gush of fresh red blood after delivery of the placenta. The seniors should be informed if the pulse rate raises by ten beats from baseline, even if the absolute rate is not alarming (above 100). After delivery, a continuous trickle of fresh blood is also a warning to inform the seniors and merits one to be proactive.

This will allow the more qualified healthcare worker to assess the case and initiate resuscitative and definitive measures to control the bleeding.

DOI: 10.1201/9781003034360-17

The number of towels/gauze pieces used, size of any clots, the blood spill on the bed/floor/ collecting units of the delivery drape help in visually estimating and quantifying the blood loss. Every labour room should display the pictorial graph as a ready reckoner. It is recommended to calculate the actual blood loss based on the number of gauze pieces/mops soaked, clots passed, or the existing collection in the collection bags.

Pictorial guidelines are available to assess blood loss objectively.

CLASSIFICATION

Based on the **temporal relation** of bleeding and delivery, it is classified as:

- **Primary PPH** that occurs at the time of delivery or within 24 hours of delivery and
- **Secondary PPH** that occurs any time after 24 hours to 6 weeks post-delivery.

Based on the *aetiology* of PPH, it is classified as:

- **Atonic**: When the uterus fails to contract after delivery, or the uterine tone remains poor. Atonicity is by far the most common cause for PPH.
- **Traumatic**: This is due to trauma to the genital tract. It can be due to briskly bleeding cervical tears, perineal tears, an extension of the episiotomy, lateral vaginal tears due to instrumental deliveries, and complete perineal tears. It is essential to realize that even a slightly higher extension of the episiotomy wound can cause significant blood loss.
- **Retained products**: Whenever there is the retention of a placental bit or membranes, it can provoke bleeding by preventing the uterus from contracting firmly. They can later get infected and cause secondary PPH also.
- **Impaired coagulation**: Even though the constriction of the arteries running across the uterine muscles is brought about by firm uterine contractions, the formation of platelet plug gets impaired at the placental delivery site. Coagulation failure, as seen in liver failure or women on anticoagulants, as well as that complicated by amniotic fluid embolism, can cause PPH.

These four causes can be remembered as the four T's (tone, trauma, tissue, and thrombosis) for ready recollection by medical students [3]

Based on the *amount of blood loss*, the PPH can be classified as

- **Minor**: 500–1,000 mL loss or
- **Major**: 1,000—1,500 mL loss.
- **Massive**: When the blood loss is more than 1,500 mL.

PREDISPOSING FACTORS

Any factor that can reduce the tone, cause trauma, increase the risk of tissue retention, or cause coagulation abnormalities are likely to cause primary PPH.

A few factors that can *cause atonicity* are:

1. Multiparity.
2. Multiple gestations.
3. Overdistension due to polyhydramnios and macrosomia.
4. Large intramural fibroid, more so when they are overlying the placental site.

5. Abruption with Couvelaire uterus: The intra-myometrial bleed in severe abruption prevents the uterus from contracting firmly. Also, there may be associated coagulation abnormalities in case of severe abruption.

6. Preterm delivery, preterm premature rupture of membranes (PPROM), and chorioamnionitis can predispose to atonic PPH if it is severe. It is because of the presence of inflammatory cells in the myometrium, the uterus fails to contract firmly.

7. The previous history of PPH is a vital predictor and warning alert.

8. Precipitate labour can be associated with atonicity.

9. Induction of labour, prolonged labour, and arrest in the second stage can cause atonicity after delivery.

10. Obesity with BMI above 40 was found to increase the risk of PPH by two-fold [4].

11. Women with pre-eclampsia are also more prone to PPH.

PREDISPOSING FACTORS FOR TRAUMA

Operative or assisted vaginal delivery, delivery of a baby with macrosomia, face to pubes delivery, precipitate labour, and unattended childbirth increase the risk of perineal tears, including complete perineal tear.

The risk of uterine rupture and or lower segment tear is higher when the caesarean section is performed late in labour, malpresentation, obstructed labour, and previously scarred uterus.

Intrauterine manipulation like the podalic version and previous uterine surgeries are also high risk for uterine rupture.

Breech delivery, prostaglandin use, and assisted vaginal birth carry the risk of cervical tears.

The factors predisposing to retaining products are abnormal placentation, chorioamnionitis, and abnormalities of the placenta.

Women with a growth-restricted fetus, previous history of curettage/manual removal of placenta, thrombophilia, and those conceived with artificial reproductive techniques have a higher likelihood of abnormal placentation. Thus, a detailed history taking and risk assessment of ongoing pregnancy can give a fair idea of those at risk for PPH. However, it can happen to any pregnant woman at delivery.

Coagulation problems need to be anticipated in women with abruption placenta, acute fatty liver of pregnancy, liver disorder and liver function derangement, thrombocytopaenia associated with HELLP (Hemolysis elevated liver enzyme and low platelet) syndrome or underlying immunologic cause. Women with chorioamnionitis, amniotic fluid embolism, and those on anticoagulants for medical disorders like mechanical heart valves are also at higher risk for bleeding. Many of the above factors might predispose to post-partum haemorrhage by more than one mechanism.

PREVENTION OF PPH

Detailed history helps in predicting the risk. In those with high risk, compatible blood should be available and kept cross-matched in the nearest blood bank. PPH should be prevented at every delivery by following universal active management of the third stage of labour (AMTSL). The following are the steps of **AMTSL**:

First step: Administration of a tocotonic agent immediately after delivery of the fetus. The pharmacological agents that can be used are

a. Intramuscular injection of 10 units of oxytocin (slow intravenous 5 units is given during caesarean section).

b. Carbetocin 100 μg intramuscular injection has been recommended recently by WHO. Carbetocin does not require a cold chain and has a longer duration of action. This makes it more suitable for countries and sets up where the cold chains cannot be ensured. At present, it is expensive and not easily affordable in peripheral centres and low-resource countries.

  c. Intravenous infusion of oxytocin drip (10 units in a 500 mL bottle of saline or ringer lactate at 30 drops per minute).
  d. Administration of misoprostol, either sublingual or oral or per rectum. Misoprostol of 600–800 µg can be administered.
  e. Hundred and fifty micrograms of prostaglandin F2α, administered intramuscularly within 1 minute of delivery of the fetus.
  f. Intravenous methyl ergometrine 0.25 mg. The administration should be timed accurately at the delivery of the anterior shoulder and followed by slow delivery of the baby to give enough time for the separated placenta to deliver out behind the fetus. Even a slight delay in administration can cause retention of the placenta due to hourglass constriction of the uterus. This drug can cause a rise in blood pressure and worsen vasospasms, so it should be used with caution.

The second step: Placenta should be delivered by controlled cord traction after observing the signs of separation of the placenta (detailed in earlier chapters).

The third step: One should feel the tone of the uterus after delivery and ensure it is contracted firmly – the WHO has recently dropped the uterine massage as a step of AMTSL.

AMTSL can reduce the risk of PPH by 60% and must be followed universally. Organization for a programme for appropriate technology in health (PATH) and WHO has advocated *Oxytocin Uniject* (is a plastic ampule containing ten units of oxytocin with a sterile needle covered by a plastic sheath that can be easily twisted and removed) for all low-resource settings. Uniject does not require injection skills and can be administered by the paramedical workers as well. In the low-resource peripheral units where uniject is not available, misoprostol must be available and used for every woman after delivery of the fetus unless contraindicated.

If the uterus doesn't feel well contracted or if the bleeding appears more than normal, the drill for the management of PPH should be initiated at the earliest in the golden first hour.

Another important aspect of prevention is ensuring that anaemia is recognized and treated during the antenatal period. Correcting anaemia will improve the capacity of the women to tolerate blood loss. The various medical disorders should be recognized and controlled with appropriate treatment in the antenatal period.

REFERENCES

  1. https://www.rcog.org.uk/en/guidelines-research-services/guidelines/gtg52/.
  2. Committee on Practice Bulletins-Obstetrics. Practice Bulletin No. 183: Postpartum hemorrhage. *Obstet Gynecol.* 2017 Oct;130(4):e168-e186. doi: 10.1097/AOG.0000000000002351. PMID: 28937571.
  3. Society of Obstetrics and Gynecology of Canada. *Post-partum haemorrhage. ALARM Manual.* The Global Library of Women's Medicine (GLOWM) 15th Ed. London 2008.
  4. Blomberg M. Maternal obesity and risk of postpartum haemorrhage. *Obstet Gynecol.* 2011 Sep. 118(3):561–568.

18 Clinical Approach to Case of PPH

Gowri Dorairajan
Jawaharlal Institute of Postgraduate Medical
Education and Research (JIPMER)

Having identified PPH, adequate resuscitation is a must. The first hour is the golden hour, and the steps taken in this hour determine the outcome. Adequate resuscitation, definitive management, and diligent monitoring should be prompt and parallel.

EFFECTIVE RESUSCITATION

The goal of resuscitation is to prevent morbidity and mortality. It is prudent to call for help. One should call the senior most of the team on-site and the consultant, if needed, early in the management. One should alert the nursing and other staff, the blood bank, and the anaesthetist. The classification of hypovolemic shock as laid down by the advanced trauma [1] life support should guide in recognizing the severity. There is a 40%–50% increase in plasma volume throughout pregnancy. One must remember that the pulse and blood pressure may show a change only when immense blood loss has happened. So, one should be alert about the visual quantification of blood loss and act accordingly. Shock index (Pulse rate/systolic blood pressure) is helpful to assess the volume loss clinically. The shock index should always be less than 1.

One should quickly secure intravenous access with a wide bore cannula (14 or 16 intravenous cannulas). If needed, two cannulae can be placed. Crystalloids should be started after taking enough blood for crossmatching and baseline haematologic profile. One must remember that colloids can interfere with crossmatching.

The foot end of the patient should be *elevated*.

Oxygen is administered by mask at 6–8 L per minute to improve tissue oxygenation.

One must remember to keep the patient *warm with a blanket or warming device* and not ignore warming because of the panic and the commotion created while resuscitating the woman. Most of the labour cots may be steel cots covered with rubber sheets, and with ongoing blood seeping on the table, the woman can start shivering due to hypothermia.

A *urinary catheter* should be inserted. The catheter not only helps improve the uterine tone by emptying the bladder but also allows one to monitor the urine output and the effectiveness of the resuscitation. The urine output should be targeted at least 30 mL/hour.

The resuscitation, monitoring, and definitive treatment must go hand in hand and parallel. Different personnel of the team working for these three aspects can achieve this goal.

- *Fluid replacement* should be sufficient to keep the systolic blood pressure above 90 mm of Hg always to prevent acute injury to other organs such as kidney and pituitary. The golden hour: the first hour is the golden hour. It is essential to recognize the volume loss and carry out an adequate fluid replacement to prevent long-term sequel and end-organ injuries as a sequel of PPH.

DOI: 10.1201/9781003034360-18

BOX 1   FIRST RESPONSE

- Call for help – Inform Senior JR/SR
  - Alert staff on duty, interns, and DRLs.
  - CCU team for CV line
  - Assess ventilator need in case of tachypnoea
- Patient in supine position/foot end elevation
- O2 by mask @ 6–8 L/min
- Secure two 16G/18G IV line
- Patient to be kept warm
- Check PR, BP, RR, and urine output

Restrict crystalloids to 2 L and initiate blood transfusion as early as possible if bleeding is not continuing. If blood is not made available by the time 2 L of crystalloids have been transfused, then another 1.5 L can be transfused as colloids. Hexa ethyl starch should be avoided. The excess volume of crystalloids carries a serious threat of dilutional coagulopathy. Pulmonary oedema can also occur if there is associated endothelial capillary dysfunction.

Blood replacement: Packed cells must be transfused if there is major blood loss. Losing 30% of blood volume can cause hemodynamic instability and shock. Blood transfusion decision is balanced to prevent shock and at the same time prevent overzealous resuscitation. The decision should be clinical and quick as the first hour (golden hour) management determines the short- and long-term outcome of the woman. Waiting for laboratory values to decide is not prudent in major blood losses, especially when the loss is continuing as lab processing takes time. Quantification of blood loss and the pulse rate and blood pressure are the most critical dictating factors for initiating blood product transfusion during major postpartum haemorrhage episodes. Blood should be crossmatched and transfused. However, crossmatching takes 30–40 minutes. To tide over this delay, group-specific blood within 15 minutes or O negative blood should be immediately available and transfused. There should be no delay in initiating blood transfusion when there is a felt need. It is better than allowing her to progress to shock or dilution coagulopathy. If blood loss exceeds 1,000 mL or tachycardia has set in (pulse rate more than 100 per minute) or the bleeding continues, then blood transfusion should be embarked on as early as possible. When four or more blood is given in 2 hours, it is a massive transfusion, and the other components need to be transfused.

Need for fresh frozen plasma (FFP) transfusion: After every six units of packed red blood cells being transfused, 4 FFP must be transfused. Further transfusion of FFP at 12–15 mL/kg (approximately 1 L FFP or four units) is needed if the prothrombin time is more than 1.5 times the control.

Platelets: It needs to be transfused if the platelet count is less than 75,000/μL and the woman is bleeding. The platelets should be targeted to be kept above 50,000/μL. Platelets should be preferable of the same group and Rh type.

Cryoprecipitate: At least two need to be transfused early in major blood loss to prevent coagulation problems. Later, if the fibrinogen level is less than 100 mg/dl, then one needs to transfuse more cryoprecipitate [2,3].

Both the FFP and cryoprecipitate should be ideally of the same group as of the woman being transfused.

Goal of blood and component replacement: Adequate and timely resuscitation with blood and components should be done to prevent hypoxia and tissue damage to any organ. The goal also is to prevent consumption coagulopathy from setting in. Therefore, the goal is to keep the Hb >8 g/dl, platelet count >75,000/μL, prothrombin time <1.5 times the control, aPTT <1.5 times the control, and fibrinogen >1 g/L.

> **BOX 2 INDICATION FOR COMPONENT TRANSFUSION**
>
> - For every 6 PC, 4 FFPs to be given.
> - If PT/a PTT >1.5 times (N), then 12–15 mL/kg or IL of FFP to be given
>
> Platelets: If counts < 50,000
> Cryo ppt: If fibrinogen <1 g/L.

Recombinant factor VIIa (rFVIIa): This can be used in life-threatening postpartum haemorrhage. However, there is limited evidence on its safety for use in obstetric haemorrhage. It has been found to increase the risk of arterial thrombosis and is usually indicated in inherited coagulopathy.

In major blood loss, *arterial blood gas analysis* (ABG) might be necessary.

Central venous line is necessary for proper fluid management to prevent fluid overload in certain patients with massive loss and high risk for pulmonary oedema due to underlying disorders, etc.

Cause directed definitive treatment should be instituted immediately along with the fluid resuscitation to stop the bleeding.

MONITORING AFTER THE INITIAL MANAGEMENT

The *vitals* like pulse, blood pressure, and oxygen saturation should be noted at the baseline and *monitored* every 15 minutes after that. If facilities exist, then one can use multiparameter monitors. After initiating the definitive management to control the bleeding, one must continue to monitor the patient. The women should be monitored for the pulse, blood pressure, respiratory rate, peripheral perfusion, urine output, mental cognition/clouding, or agitation (suggestive of cerebral hypoxia) every half hour for the next 2 hours. When she has been stabilized, it can be relaxed to every hour. If multiparameter monitors are available, then continuous monitoring of the same should be done.

One needs to collect the investigations sent and assess for any derangements and continue to monitor the coagulation profile, platelet count, kidney function (urea and creatinine), and hemogram after 4 hours. Monitoring of the ABG may be necessary for a woman who had massive PPH/tachypnoea or decreased level of consciousness.

In women who have received more than 1.5 L of crystalloids, whose urine output is less than 30 mL per hour, and who have undergone prolonged surgery, central venous pressure (CVP) should guide the fluid replacement.

Communication: It is the caregiver's responsibility to inform the woman and her relatives about the fact that there is PPH. The caregivers should periodically inform the woman's condition, bleeding status, and the components transfused to the woman and the relatives.

Emotional support to the woman is also an integral part of the management. The woman should also be taken into confidence about the plan and periodically informed about her progress.

Complications of PPH: These include

- Haemorrhagic hypovolemic shock
- Acute kidney injury
- Consumption coagulopathy
- Acute respiratory distress syndrome
- Sheehan syndrome
- Multiorgan failure
- Sepsis
- Uterine necrosis following compression sutures
- Thromboembolism

BOX 3   MONITORING A WOMAN WITH PPH

1. Assess every 15 minutes in the acute bleeding phase every 30 minutes to 1 hour afterwards.
   a. Pulse rate
   b. Blood pressure
   c. Respiratory rate
   d. Peripheral perfusion
   e. Urine output
   f. Mental cognition Clouding or agitation may suggest hypotension/hypoxia)
2. Investigation:
   Collect the investigation reports end at the time of diagnosis as early as possible
   a. Assess for features suggestive of DIC
   b. Monitor coagulation parameters
   c. Hemogram
   d. Renal function test
   e. ABG, especially in the presence of massive haemorrhage/tachypnoea/decreased level of consciousness
3. Invasive monitoring:
   Early CVP line insertion may guide in fluid resuscitation/replacement (Cautious in the presence of suspected DIC)

- Operative intervention, hysterectomy, and ureteric injury
- Massive blood transfusion and related complications such as haemolysis and acute lung injury (TALLY)
- Maternal death

Massive blood transfusion, surgical management of PPH, intubation, and ventilation add to various specific complications related to them.

DEFINITIVE MANAGEMENT

Ascertaining the cause: As mentioned earlier, there are four major causes. To know which is the cause in the index case, one needs to know the type of delivery, especially if it was an instrument-assisted delivery.

The steps to ascertain the cause are to

Feel with the left hand on the sterile drape if the uterus is midline and well contracted. If the uterus feels flabby, it is most likely atonic PPH. If the uterus contracts and relaxes in between with a gush of bleeding, one should also rule out retained placenta or membranes. One should examine the placenta and membranes for missing cotyledons and missing portions of the membrane.

A digital examination should be done to feel for any membrane bits or placental bit in the internal os and, if present, can be digitally removed.

One should do any further exploration by hand or instrument in the uterine cavity to remove retained products with some form of anaesthesia. Intravenous sedation in the labour room is the least that one should offer. The retained bits should be removed digitally or with ovum forceps. A sticky membrane that is not getting pulled out might need gentle curettage with a blunt curette or the anterior vaginal wall retractor. These procedures are attended by the severe risk of neurogenic shock, sepsis, and uterine perforation. Due precautions should be taken, and one has to be gentle. Tocotonics are used as the uterine cavity is getting emptied to ensure a firmly contracted uterus.

In women where the abdominal examination reveals a firmly contracted uterus, but brisk fresh bleeding is going on, there is reason to suspect trauma to the genital tract even in the absence of any assisted vaginal birth.

Examination to detect trauma to the genital tract: In cases suspected to have trauma, a systematic approach must be followed. It should be done under good light with reasonable assistance. Intravenous sedation is essential to gain cooperation from the woman, especially when the bleeding is brisk, and time is a critical factor for managing the tears. If needed, the exploration and suturing are done in the operation theatre under anaesthesia. Anaesthesia gives an advantage of a thorough job, and the fact that the woman is being monitored and resuscitated by the anaesthetist provides a benefit to the surgeon to focus on the tears and suturing. The resuscitation should continue till she is taken to the operation theatre, and a pack in the vagina would reduce bleeding by the pressure effect.

Exploration of the cervix (Figure 18.1a and b):
Exploration of the cervix needs two Sims speculums, three sponge holdings, or ring forceps.

One Sim's speculum is used to retract the posterior vaginal wall. The other is used to retract the anterior vaginal wall. The cervix is held with a ring forceps at 12 o'clock position. Depending on how frilly the cervix is, another ring forceps is applied at 2 or 3 o'clock position. A third ring forceps is applied at 4 or 6 o'clock position. The cervix is visualized for intactness between 12 and 3 o'clock and 3 and 6 o'clock segments. Then the ring forceps from 3 o'clock is moved to 8 or 9 o'clock position. The segment between 6 and 8 o'clock is examined for intactness. The 12 o'clock ring forceps are not moved to mark the starting and the endpoint of the examination. This is also described as walking around the cervix to look for any tears.

Exploration of the lower tract: After cleaning and draping the woman, the perineum is examined for any tear or extension of the episiotomy by visualizing the apex. Any bleeders should be quickly clamped with a haemostatic clamp or artery forceps. The vagina should be methodically and thoroughly examined with the help of digital and speculum-aided retraction. Starting from the episiotomy site, one can look for an apex extension upwards to the midline and anal sphincter complex. Gradually, explore laterally away from the episiotomy for satellite tears, including pocket tears in the lateral vagina and spiral tears from the lateral vagina to the fornix. Continue the examination to the opposite side. One should examine all the fornices till the cervical reflection to rule out any hidden high-up tears. The paraurethral regions should be examined for any tears.

Per rectal examination should be done to feel for rectal mucosa and the internal and external sphincter by pill-rolling movement. Button-hole tears involving the rectum with intact perineum should also be excluded.

One must make a note of all the various tears before suturing begins. Reexploring or exploring higher up after a few sutures are taken in the lower vagina places the already sutured area under serious threat of disruption due to the handling and stretching. So, one must always follow two dictums:

- Do not explore for tears higher up after partial suturing or after initiating suturing in the lower aspect.
- Start suturing the highest tear first (cervical tear before vaginal tear and higher vaginal tears) before suturing the lower tear or episiotomy or complete perineal tear.

Vaginal digital examination also would reveal any blood collecting in the paravaginal tissues. The blood may escape from the apex, or any bleeder may bleed submucosally in the pocket created by the tear.

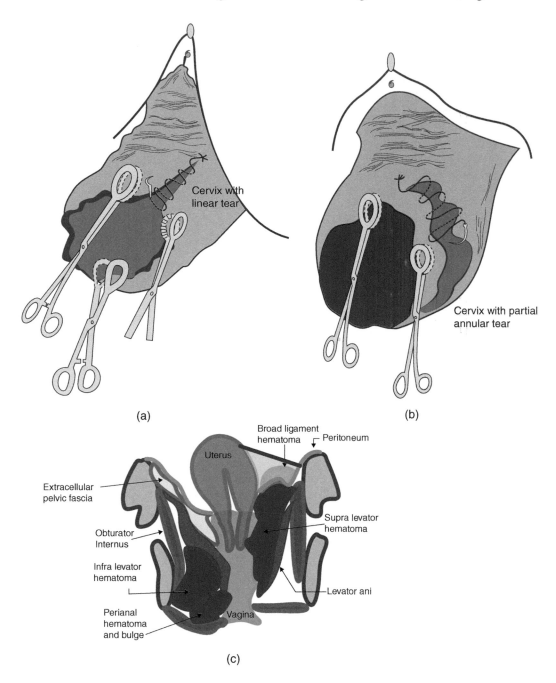

(a)

(b)

(c)

FIGURE 18.1 (a) The exploration of the cervix with three-ring forceps revealing linear tear with suture placement. (b) Line diagram showing partial annual tear on the cervix and placement of suture. (c) Line diagram showing vaginal hematoma. Supralevator hematoma can extend as broad ligament hematoma.

A digital bimanual examination to rule **broad ligament hematoma** is necessary when the uterus is not midline and the maternal condition is deteriorating (tachycardia and fall in blood pressure and increasing pallor) out of proportion to the revealed blood loss. Any soft or firm swelling felt to the side of the uterus through the fornices or through rectal examination should make us suspect broad ligament haematoma.

Usually, hematomas are likely to form a few hours after delivery or suturing of the tears. When a high cervical tear has been missed, or the bleeder at the apex of the tear had retracted and did not get included in the ligature, the risk of broad ligament haematoma increases. Broad ligament hematomas are also possible in some cases of previous scar dehiscence or intrapartum rupture near the lateral uterine wall. Post-delivery retraction of the uterus reduces the briskness of the bleeding. Slow ooze may continue to cause hemoperitoneum of broad ligament hematoma.

Vaginal hematomas: These are hematomas that usually form in the lateral vaginal wall (paravaginal hematomas). These can be infralevator or supralevator (Figure 18.1c). The supra levator can expand towards the extraperitoneal pelvic cellular tissue and extend towards the broad ligament. These hematomas may not present as vulval swelling. They are felt on vaginal and rectal examination as swelling in the paravaginal area in the middle or superior aspect depending on its location to the levator ani muscle. Some of these can be very expansile holding up to 500 mL of blood and can cause features of hypovolemia.

Vulvo-vaginal hematomas: These hematomas are seen as outward swelling at the vulva.

These haematomata can form due to a retracted blood vessel in the layers of the episiotomy that escaped the ligature.

They are recognized by a shiny blue/purple swelling stretching the vulva, commonly at the episiotomy site. The vulval hematomas may be associated with hematomas extending upwards along the lateral vaginal wall, submucosally, or in the paravaginal plane.

REFERENCES

1. American College of Surgeons Committee on Trauma. *Advanced Trauma Life Support for Doctors– Student Course Manual*. 8th ed. Chicago: American College of Surgeons; 2008.
2. https://www.rcog.org.uk/en/guidelines-research-services/guidelines/gtg52/.
3. https://www.rcog.org.uk/globalassets/documents/guidelines/gtg-47.pdf.

19 Specific Management of PPH

Gowri Dorairajan
Jawaharlal Institute of Postgraduate Medical
Education and Research (JIPMER)

MANAGEMENT OF ATONIC POSTPARTUM HAEMORRHAGE

If the bleeding is due to an atonic uterus, the following needs to be done for the definitive treatment immediately.

1. *Catheterise the bladder* if not already done. Emptying the bladder improves uterine contraction and tone. It also gives access to monitor the urine output.
2. *Starting pharmacological agents* to bring about uterine contractions include the following.
   a. Administer ten units of oxytocin intramuscularly if not administered for prevention of PPH.
   b. Starting oxytocin infusion through a drip of 10 units in a 500 mL ringer lactate bottle started at 30 drops per minute.
   c. Two hundred and fifty micrograms prostaglandin F2α can be administered through intramuscular injection. We can repeat the same every 15 minutes up to 8 injections theoretically. However, the author believes that if two such injections have not worked, then it is time to be more proactive and consider surgical management. In addition, these injections can bring about diarrhoea and vomiting that can worsen hypovolemia.
   d. Inject methyl ergometrine 0.25 mg administered intravenously. If the uterus has not contracted even after this injection, one can repeat it as an intramuscular injection once. Theoretically, one can administer up to five times, but the author believes that additional doses are not likely to work if two have not worked. Therefore, one should be proactive for surgical management instead of wasting the golden hour with repeated doses as they may not work.
   e. If none of these is readily available or has not worked, then 600 to up to 1,000 µg of misoprostol can be used. It can be inserted rectally or given orally.
   f. Tranexamic acid is recommended for all cases of postpartum haemorrhage. It is not recommended for prevention. The WHO recommends its use in all cases of PPH irrespective of the cause. However, it should be given within 3 hours of childbirth. It is administered as a fixed dose of 1 g in 10 mL (100 mg/mL) intravenously, at 1 mL per minute. A second dose is recommended if bleeding continues after 30 minutes.
3. While administering these pharmacological agents, the obstetrician should initiate *external massage of the uterus*. Initiate *bimanual massage* as soon as possible as it gives better compression than external massage (Figure 19.1a).
4. If the woman bleeds due to atonicity *despite the above measures, then one should embark upon surgical management* in the theatre. The decision for mobilising to the theatre depends on the amount of bleed, the pulse rate, blood pressure, and response to the above measures. There is no hard and fast rule. In general, if the above steps have not worked, the decision should be taken in an hour. One should take an earlier decision if she is bleeding briskly and there is no response whatsoever to the above measures.
5. *Alternate non-surgical options*

DOI: 10.1201/9781003034360-19

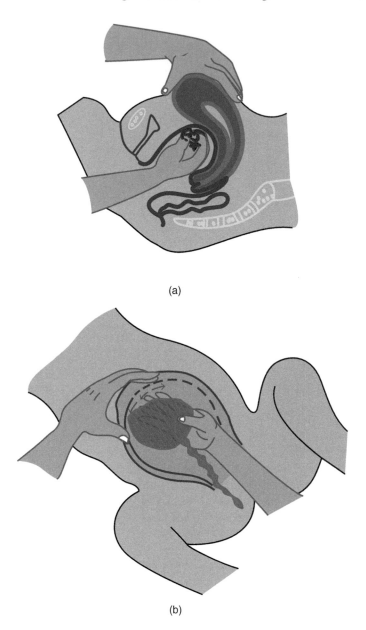

(a)

(b)

FIGURE 19.1   (a) Line diagram depicting bimanual massage for atonic uterus. (b) Line diagram showing technique of manual removal of placenta.

Balloon tamponade is a procedure that involves inflating the uterine cavity with a durable and stretchable balloon to arrest bleeding by pressure. It has a balloon tied to one end of a catheter. The balloon end of the catheter is inserted in the uterus and inflated. One must remember that the flabby puerperal uterus has an immense capacity, and the inflation needs to be voluminous enough to cause pressure. The author feels that the balloon inflation should be used as a temporary measure while transporting the woman to a facility with expertise and a replete blood bank or in the tertiary hospital as one awaits uterine artery embolisation procedure. *Bakri Balloon,* approved by the FDA for this purpose, is made of silicon. It has a dual channel. One is the inflation port for inflating the uterus and the other is the drainage port for measuring blood loss. It must be inflated to 500 mL.

The Rusch urological balloon, Sengstaken Blakemore oesophageal catheter, and Condom catheter have all been used. A tamponade test helps to confirm that the balloon system will work in the woman [1,2].

Uterine artery clamp has been recently studied for occluding the uterine arteries. It is applied with one blade on the cervix and the other on the lateral vaginal fornix and clamped to occlude the uterine artery. There is a serious risk of trauma and occlusion of the ureter, and the author does not advocate this to the postgraduates.

Recently a vacuum-induced device called *JADA device* [3] to control bleeding has been studied. The device creates a vacuum in the uterine cavity. The suction brings the two walls together and opposes the walls giving the squeeze effect and reducing blood loss.

Uterine artery embolisation can be performed by catheters placed in the arteries from the femoral artery. This procedure can serve as an alternative to laparotomy and ligation of vessels. The infrastructure must be available in the emergency hour. Preferably the uterine artery, alternatively, the internal iliac arteries, if the uterine artery could not be accessed, can be embolised with silicone gel material with the help of the Waltman loop. The procedure is performed under fluoroscopy or ultrasound guidance. The significant problems with these procedures are uterine necrosis and deep vein thrombosis. Hemoperitoneum might occur while approaching the internal iliac arteries during the process of negotiation into the vessels.

The traditional surgical options are always quick and rewarding to control bleeding. Every obstetrician should be well versed in these procedures.

STEPWISE SURGICAL DEVASCULARISATION

The decision for surgical intervention should be taken for atonic PPH not responding to the pharmacological agents mentioned above. The golden hour is the first hour. If the bleeding is not controlled, then adequate resuscitation should go on, and the patient prepared for surgical intervention. Ensure that sufficient blood and components are available. One should not allow a patient to slip from grade 1 to 3 of shock before surgical management; otherwise, there will be irreversible organ injury despite surgical intervention. Trying non-surgical options without previous experience or in the absence of suitable devices amounts to wasting time and allowing the haemodynamic condition to worsen.

The principles of surgical intervention

The surgical intervention is always done under general anaesthesia.

The abdomen is opened by a vertical midline sub-umbilical incision. If surgical intervention is required for excess bleeding within a few hours of a caesarean section performed by a suprapubic transverse incision, then the same incision can be taken.

The first step after opening the abdomen is to observe for any free fluid, abnormal smell, and hemoperitoneum. One should examine the uterus, the previous scar site if relevant, and the broad ligament for any pathologies. One should note the tone of the uterus. One should also rule out any broad ligament haematoma.

Compression sutures: If the patient had a vaginal delivery, then a Hayman suture should be applied. If the atonic PPH was at the time of the caesarean section, then one can choose to do uterine artery ligation first and then proceed with B-lynch compression sutures.

Necessary precautions are that the compression suture should *never involve needle bites of the upper segment*. No modified sutures involving the upper part should be attempted. In this regard, the author would like to quote a case.

Case: This case is before the B-lynch suture became the standard protocol. A woman was admitted at 34 weeks with severe preeclampsia, abruption, and intrauterine death. Labour was induced, and the women delivered a stillborn fetus. There were significant retroplacental clots. A massive atonic postpartum haemorrhage followed the delivery. The uterus did not respond to pharmacological agents, so surgical intervention was carried out. Systematic devascularisation was done, and in a desperate attempt to save the uterus, a figure of 8 compression suture was applied in the upper segment of the myometrium and was tied tightly. The suture controlled the bleeding. The patient successfully recovered after intensive support and massive blood and component transfusion. One year later, she presented at 24 weeks of pregnancy in haemorrhagic shock with intrauterine death and hemoperitoneum. Urgent laparotomy was performed. At laparotomy, there was a 1-L hemoperitoneum. The upper segment of the uterus had ruptured in a Z shape at the site of the previous compression suture. A hysterectomy was performed.

It is essential to understand that women with needle bites in the upper segment of the uterus for modified compression sutures have a severe risk of uterine rupture in the subsequent pregnancy.

The other precaution is that *absorbable suture* like catgut 1 is used to apply compression sutures. Braided suture like polyglactin should be avoided. It can act as a saw on the uterine wall when it is tightened, disrupt the myometrium, and again pose the risk of rupture of the uterus at this weak myometrial portion in the subsequent pregnancy.

Uterine artery ligature: It is done at the level of the internal os at the lateral wall of the uterus. The uterine vessels start ascending at that level. A deep bite, including the lower lateral wall to occlude the uterine artery, is the safest and quickest procedure. One need not necessarily skeletonise the uterine artery to ligate it. Either absorbable sutures like catgut or delayed absorbable polyglactin are used for uterine artery ligation. The uterine branch of the ovarian artery is ligated at the cornual end below the fallopian tube, with a suture passed to include a part of the adjoining uterine wall. This O'Leary ligature occludes the uterine branch coming down from the ovarian vessels via the mesosalpinx.

Internal iliac artery ligation [4]: Bilateral internal iliac artery ligation reduces the pulse pressure by 85% and the blood flow by 50% and can drastically reduce the bleeding. However, many collaterals with deep femoral arteries and the ovarian arteries rescue the blood supply and prevent ischaemic damage to other organs. It is a necessary procedure when one is desperate to preserve the uterus. It needs expertise as well as takes time and reasonable assistance for proper exposure. The retroperitoneum is exposed by pulling the uterus anteriorly and to the opposite side. The posterior peritoneum over the psoas major muscle between the round ligament and the infundibulopelvic ligament is incised. The incision is extended longitudinally until the pelvic brim parallel to the infundibulopelvic ligament, keeping the ureter in the medial flap. Identify the bifurcation of the common iliac artery. The internal iliac artery is inferiomedial as it enters the pelvis. The external iliac artery continues laterally along with the psoas muscle.

The internal iliac artery is ligated with the help of right-angled artery forceps. One must be careful of the internal iliac vein running inferiomedial to the artery and the external iliac vein running inferior and lateral while driving the right-angled forceps underneath the internal iliac artery from lateral to the medial side. The ligation should be done 4 cm below the origin of the internal iliac artery so that the anterior division is ligated and the posterior division is spared. The posterior division gives parietal branches.

Suppose there is brisk bleed and circulatory collapse even while opening the abdomen. In such a situation, an assistant compresses the aorta as the first step on opening the abdomen, and the chief surgeon proceeds with hysterectomy or devascularisation.

A clamp covered with rubber tubing can be placed on the infundibulopelvic ligament and released intermittently till a definitive procedure is completed to arrest the bleeding.

Caesarean hysterectomy is considered the fastest and most definitive treatment for atonic haemorrhage among women in shock.

If the woman is multiparous and has already had massive PPH, then it may be prudent to accomplish caesarean hysterectomy (subtotal) instead of internal iliac ligation. Subtotal caesarean hysterectomy can be completed extremely fast.

Since the pedicles are likely to be engorged, enlarged, and oedematous, cutting between three clamps (keeping two clamps lateral and one medial) will prevent calamity due to slipping clamps.

One need not waste time taking the round ligament separately. The fundal structures can be taken as one structure to include the fallopian tube, the ovarian ligament, and the round ligament. The bladder needs to be pushed down. The broad ligament might need progressive clamps. Uterine arteries can be once again ligated at the level of the internal os. Subtotal hysterectomy would suffice in cases of atonic PPH if the placenta was not previa.

Antibiotics, blood component replacement, and intensive supportive therapy usually result in complete recovery without any long-term sequel.

Thromboprophylaxis is administered in selected cases with an underlying risk of thrombosis. It is started only when we are sure that there is no thrombocytopenia or ongoing coagulopathy. Compression stockings and early ambulation are other measures to prevent thrombosis.

MANAGEMENT OF TRAUMATIC PPH

Whenever trauma is suspected, the genital tract is explored for any trauma, as detailed in the previous chapter. The tears detected need to be sutured.

- **Suturing of cervical tear**
  - **Linear tears**: The edges of the cervical tear are held with ring forceps. The apex should be well visualised. The suturing should begin above the apex. Interrupted sutures with absorbable material like catgut 0 or catgut 1 are preferred. Braided sutures like polyglactin can increase the risk of infection, and they can also cut through in friable tissues.
    - The sutures can be simple or mattresses depending on the bleeding and the friability of the margins.
    - If the apex is high and cannot be visualised, then one can suture at the highest visualised margin and keep a stay on that suture to give traction. With traction, subsequent higher sutures can be taken till one reaches beyond the apex.
    - Small tears, even if not bleeding, should be sutured to prevent ectropion and incompetent cervix in the future.
  - **Annular tears**: Sometimes, there can be avulsion of a whole ring of the cervix with only a flimsy attachment to the cervix. This is more often seen following vacuum extraction before full dilation. The cervical lips get caught within the vacuum cup and tear. Such a detached portion of the cervix should be sutured if the cervix looks pink by interrupted or continuous sutures back to the main cervix. If, however, it is completely detached and the detached portion is black or friable, suturing back the detached bit may be difficult. In such a situation blanket interlocking suture at the edge of the raw cervix should be given to ensure haemostasis of the raw edge of the cervix.
  - **Bucket handle tear**: This is a condition when a part of the cervix gets avulsed circularly while the majority of the cervix is intact (Figure 18.1c Chapter 18). This tear can be easily sutured back to the cervix by either continuous or interrupted sutures. Bucket handle tears are likely after vacuum extraction as well as a complication of the use of prostaglandin F2α for second-trimester abortions.
- **Vaginal tears**
  - **Linear tears**: Linear tears of the vagina are likely to happen more so in the lateral walls of the vagina. These are to be adequately visualised and stitched separately from the episiotomy. It can be sutured as continuous or interrupted simple sutures to ensure haemostasis and obliterate dead space.
  - **Pocket tears**: These are spiral tears. They can be in the lateral wall and spiral up to the fornix. These tears are likely to be deep and are associated with deep separation of paravaginal tissue much deeper and away from the margins of the tear. They are likely to form haematoma if not recognised well. The suturing involves obliterating the dead

space with a separate suture before stitching the margins of the tears. The tear edges are approximated with continuous or interrupted stitches, preferably with non-braided absorbable material like catgut 0 or 1.

- **Tears involving fornix**: These are difficult to suture as they are high up. It should be sutured under good light and with good exposure. If need be, it can be sutured under complete anaesthesia. The spiral lateral wall tears that have extended up to the lateral fornix can pose a serious threat to the ureter while suturing as the ureter is within 2 cm from the lateral fornix. These tears can be approximated by interrupted sutures with absorbable non-braided suture material.

- **Extension of the episiotomy apex**: sometimes, the apex of the episiotomy can extend high up to involve the fornix. One must visualise the apex and start suturing about a centimetre above the apex. It might be necessary to pack the cervix away to visualise the apex of the tear. The packing is done with a medium-size tailed tampon with the tail coming out of the vagina. The cervix may have to be retracted up with the blade of the Sims speculum to visualise the apex of the tear. The principle of suturing remains the same, as mentioned earlier. Dead space must be obliterated if needed by separate sutures running below and behind the torn edges before the edges are closed off.

Satellite tears should be sutured separately.

Sometimes it may be prudent to leave a roller gauze pack in the vagina to give pressure even after suturing the tear. The insertion of the pack should be done gently with lubrication to prevent abrasion of the vagina while packing.

Suturing of complete perineal tears [5]: The extent of the tear should be identified by per rectal and combined rectal, vaginal examination before proceeding with suturing. Pill rolling movement helps in delineating the loss of the internal sphincter layer. It also helps in detecting external sphincter tear and its extent. One can also make out any extension to the anal or the rectal mucosa by rectal examination.

One should classify the perineal tears as per the Sultan Classification [6].

The anal mucosa is sutured with polyglactin 30. The recent recommendation is that the suture can be submucosal alone without penetrating the lumen. It can be a continuous suture. Earlier catgut was used, and the mucosa was sutured with interrupted suture with knots in the rectal lumen. The suturing starts well above the apex. A second layer should identify and include the internal sphincter, which is again taken as a continuous suture. The internal anal sphincter is preferably sutured as an end-to-end mattress with delayed absorbable suture.

The external anal sphincter tends to retract because of the high basal tone, especially when it is completely torn. The retracted end should be identified and held with Allis forceps.

The partial tear can be sutured by end-to-end repair with a mattress suture across the two partially torn ends. The delayed absorbable sutures are preferable for the sphincters.

If the tear is complete (stage 3b), then the overlapping technique is preferred. The whole sphincter complex should be well-identified and held, and mobilised a little to suture by overlapping. Once the anal mucosa and the sphincter complex are sutured, then the superficial and deep perineal muscles should be sutured with interrupted sutures. The vaginal mucosa should be approximated with catgut. This is followed by suturing of the perineal skin either by the mattress or subcuticular absorbable suture.

Before suturing the complete perineal tear, administering a prophylactic dose of antibiotic (ceftriaxone 1 gm) is recommended. Foley's catheter may be inserted for 12 hours. Stool softeners like lactulose or liquid paraffin 15 mL two to three times a day are administered for 7–10 days. Pelvic floor and sphincter exercises are recommended after 7 days.

MANAGEMENT OF RETAINED PRODUCTS

When the delivered placenta or the membranes are incomplete, or there was a difficulty, and the placenta was removed piecemeal, then one should suspect retained products as the cause for the bleeding. There may be occasions when the placenta fails to deliver spontaneously, and the woman starts bleeding. In such a situation, manual removal of the placenta might be necessary. In these situations, the placental adhesion is at the level of the decidua only. However, they fail to separate spontaneously. They easily separate with mechanical shearing force at the basal plate.

Manual removal of the placenta: This is performed under general anaesthesia in the operation theatre. In women where the placenta did not separate despite tocotonics and there is no associated bleeding, we need to be alert about the possibility of placenta accreta. If the woman is not bleeding, we can look at the previous records for comment on placental adherence, and if needed, one can do ultrasonography to rule out accreta before proceeding.

MRP is contraindicated in known placenta accrete or higher grade adhesion syndromes.

Under all aseptic precautions, in the operation theatre, the procedure is carried out in a lithotomy position. A cupped right gloved hand is introduced into the vagina. The fingers follow the cord to reach the placental site (Figure 19.1b). The fingers are insinuated at the placental edge between the basal plate and the decidua while the thumb remains at the cord site – the left hand steadies the uterus by grabbing the fundus of the uterus through the abdominal wall externally. The fingers inside provide the mechanical force to shear the placental attachment from the decidua and are moved from side to side as they are advanced from the margin towards the bulk till the other margin of the placenta. Once the placenta is separated, it is grabbed in hand and delivered. One should inform the anaesthetists to stop the uterine relaxation and start tocotonics. Once the placenta is delivered, check for its completeness.

Ensure that the uterus is contracted well and there is no postpartum bleed. Sometimes, the placenta may be superficially adherent and is removed piecemeal. Excessive bleeding can follow. One should avoid undue force to pull any adherent bit. Instead, it can be left behind as there may be focal accrete. If bits have been left behind, then therapeutic antibiotics should be given. Levels of β-hCG might have to be monitored if a major chunk is left behind. The endpoint of the procedure of MRP for such adherence placenta could be stoppage of bleeding rather than an overzealous attempt at instrumental evacuation to ensure complete removal. The latter can be attended by continued bleeding requiring further measure, including possible hysterectomy.

The remaining placental bit is likely to get expelled spontaneously within a few days. One must be vigilant for secondary haemorrhage and sepsis.

To conclude, the definitive management is directed towards the cause. Effective resuscitation, identification of the cause, and the definitive treatment must go on as a parallel process. The resuscitation goals must be kept in mind, and the definitive treatment should be able to succeed in the arrest of bleeding, failing which decision for surgical intervention including hysterectomy should be taken before the woman sustains irreversible organ damage due to haemorrhage.

Postoperative care of PPH in the high dependency unit or obstetric ICU should focus on multiorgan function monitoring and supportive care. These women are more prone to acute kidney injury, sepsis, thromboembolism, and coagulation problems.

Respiratory support, intravenous fluids, broad-spectrum antibiotics, compression stockings, and anticoagulants after 12 hours of surgery are usually necessary for woman requiring surgical methods to arrest bleeding. Clinical evaluation and biochemical and haematological evaluation are required periodically to monitor for other end-organ dysfunction.

One must watch for unusual complications depending on the procedure carried out: gluteal region pain in internal iliac ligation, uterine necrosis in compression suture along with devascularisation, urine leak in women with difficult caesarean hysterectomy mainly when performed in the setting of placenta previa/accreta syndrome, and endocrine organ failure due to Sheehan syndrome

SECONDARY POSTPARTUM HAEMORRHAGE

This condition is defined as the occurrence of excessive or abnormal bleeding from the uterus after 24 hours and till 12 weeks postpartum. It occurs in about 0.5%–1% of pregnancies. The causes include endometritis, retained products, placental polyp, gestational trophoblastic disease, placental site trophoblastic tumour, and arteriovenous malformation (AVM). Rarely coagulation abnormality due to evolving liver disorder, anticoagulant intake, immunologic thrombocytopaenia, haematological malignancies, and fibroid polyp needs to be kept in mind.

PPH is more often associated with subclinical endometritis compared to frank sepsis.

The clinical evaluation should include the history of the type of delivery, any problems in the second or third stage, and any risk factors for retaining bits of the placenta as enumerated previously should also be evaluated. The woman is likely to be anaemic. The uterus is expected to be sub-involuted and slightly tender. There may be a fresh bleed from the vagina. The bleed may be associated with a foul smell if the problem manifests after a few days of birth.

Management includes supportive therapy with intravenous fluids and blood and components depending on the amount of blood loss and the condition of the woman.

Evaluation mandates ultrasonography to diagnose retained products inside the uterine cavity. The same might be identified as a placental polyp. Doppler studies need to be done to rule out gestational trophoblastic disease and AVM. Serum βhCG may be necessary in cases with suspicion of gestational trophoblastic disease. Most of the AVMs are acquired.

Episodic torrential bleeds can happen with acquired AVM of the uterine artery. Inflammation, infection, and recent caesarean section in the advanced stage of labour can also result in AV malformation.

The condition of the woman needs to be evaluated by noting down the pulse, blood pressure, and pallor besides the specific evaluation mentioned above.

Other investigations include cervical swab and blood cultures, haematological evaluation for type and severity of anaemia as well as a peripheral smear for any abnormal cells. It is necessary to evaluate coagulation profile and liver function. Angiography would be required to confirm an AVM and treat it by embolisation at the same setting if feasible.

Treatment: The mainstay is broad-spectrum antibiotics along with resuscitation and blood and component replacement depending on the volume of loss. Antibiotics should target gram-positive as well as negatives and anaerobes (for example, a combination of clindamycin and gentamycin). If the woman is bleeding heavily and there are retained products, surgical evacuation is indicated. It should be preferably attempted under anaesthesia in the operation theatre after a shot of antibiotics. Suppose the bleeding is not very heavy and the woman is stable. In that case, the evacuation can be postponed to an elective hour after a course of antibiotics and after building up her haemoglobin. Surgical evacuation is fraught with increased risk of perforation as well increased bleeding. It should be carried out gently by an experienced member of the team. Rarely, the bleeding might get exaggerated and might require balloon tamponing or devascularisation.

Preparation for uterine artery embolisation can be undertaken before elective evacuation, depending on the availability.

The arteriovenous malformation can be managed conservatively with antibiotics and component therapy if the bleeding is not excessive. Blood and component transfusion is necessary to build up the haemoglobin. These women are likely to have episodic bleeding. Uterine artery or internal iliac artery embolisation through the femoral artery can be electively planned. Ultimately, if the bleeding becomes torrential and does not respond to or if the procedure of embolisation fails, then hysterectomy may be resorted to for stopping torrential bleed for cases of acquired AVM. Rarely direct injection to embolise the AVM has been tried to conserve the uterus.

MASSIVE BLOOD TRANSFUSION

It refers to a situation when ten units of blood have been transfused in 24 hours or when one entire blood volume has been replaced in 24 hours, or 50% of blood volume is replaced within 3 hours.

A retrospective diagnosis after 24 hours carries less clinical value when there is a scenario of ongoing blood loss. Therefore, transfusion of 4 units within 1 hour can be taken as a working definition to follow the protocol of massive transfusion to prevent the onset of coagulopathy and acidosis.

Transfusion of packed red blood cells, plasma, and platelet are likely to maintain the composition of the transfused fluid close to that of blood.

Massive transfusion protocol should be observed in every centre that deals with cases with massive blood loss. All blood banks should maintain massive transfusion packages, and once activated or sounded, the correct proportion of all compatible products should be made available in the shortest time. Thus, save time spent on individual product compatibility testing.

The ratio usually followed in obstetrics is 1:1:1. That means for every four packed red blood cells transfused within 2 hours, equal units of fresh frozen plasma and platelets should be empirically transfused. Many hospitals follow the 3:2:2 ratio for obstetric haemorrhage due to the pregnancy-related changes in the coagulation system.

Inadequate perfusion causes shock, which leads to acidosis, endothelial damage, and systemic inflammatory response. The endothelial damage can trigger intravascular binding of platelets and fibrinogen, thereby causing intravascular coagulopathy, which further depletes the available platelets and fibrinogen to arrest bleeding.

Overzealous perfusion with crystalloids or packed red blood cells alone can bring about increased hydrostatic pressure at the capillary level and result in interstitial oedema as well as dilutional coagulopathy due to infusion of fluids deficient in coagulation factors.

Other problems of massive transfusion include hypothermia, which is a serious problem if the blood and products are not warmed. There can be an increase in levels of potassium and citrate and a decrease in magnesium levels.

Targets of massive transfusion: Besides the haematological targets mentioned in this chapter the other targets are to maintain a body temperature above 35° centigrade, maintain pH of blood between 7.3 and 7.4, and base deficit less than 2 meq/L.

COAGULOPATHY AND ITS MANAGEMENT

Coagulopathy is a challenging problem in obstetrics. The cause is inherited coagulation factor deficiency, postpartum haemorrhage, obstetric problems like abruption, placental adhesive syndrome, amniotic fluid embolism, severe sepsis causing systemic inflammation, acute fatty liver of pregnancy, and liver failure due to hepatitis. Massive blood transfusion and anticoagulant therapy can also cause coagulopathy.

The cause of disseminated intravascular coagulation and consumption coagulopathy in obstetrics is diverse.

Screening in pregnancy: There is an increase in coagulation factors, plasma volume, and decreased platelet count and RBC mass in pregnancy. The best screening test in pregnancy is a thorough history seeking excess menstrual bleed, an easy tendency to bruises, gum bleed, and family history of bleeding predisposition. In the absence of any forthcoming history, further lab screening is not necessary. Low platelet counts are reflective of a propensity for bleeding in pregnancy.

The profile in suspected cases includes prothrombin time, activated partial thromboplastin, and platelet count. In the obstetric setting of bleeding, especially in abruption and severe preeclampsia, bedside point of care clot retraction time helps in knowing the capacity to clot and the ability of clot to retract to leave clear serum within 30 minutes of clotting. When the blood does not clot well or does not leave behind clear serum, one should suspect that there is ongoing fibrinolysis where the clot retraction does not leave behind clear serum. Fibrin production can be indirectly measured by assessing the levels of fibrin degradation product D-Dimer. Fibrinogen level assay also reflects DIC, though it is less specific. Fibrinogen levels give clinical guidance to the component transfusion. Thromboelastography (TEG) is an objective method of studying coagulation, but the experience of its use in obstetrics haemorrhage is limited in the literature.

Known coagulation disorder: If the woman and the caregiver are aware of an underlying know coagulation problem, then the specific levels should be checked in the first and second trimester and later at 34–36 weeks and kept corrected. The factors should be transfused close to the delivery to avert bleeding if the levels of the affected component are low. Idiopathic thrombocytopenic purpura is a common condition encountered in pregnancy. A target platelet above 50,000 during pregnancy is a safe target. Platelets should be at least 20,000 for vaginal delivery and 80,000 for safe outcomes after caesarean section. Neuraxial anaesthesia mandates a count of 75,000.

Known use of anticoagulation: The woman may be on anticoagulants due to underlying problems like a prosthetic valve and acquired or inherited thrombophilias. The vitamin antagonists should be changed to unfractionated heparin or enoxaparin at term. At the onset of labour, the subsequent doses should be skipped and resumed 6–12 hours after child birth depending on the mode of delivery. Antidotes like protamine sulfate should be stocked and used if the delivery is impending within 6 hours of the last dose of heparin. Fresh frozen plasma and platelet transfusion might be needed in the wake of excessive bleeding or if the women came in labour before switching over from vitamin antagonists like the coumarin group of drugs.

Obstetric factors: Underlying antepartum haemorrhage due to abruption and placenta previa can predispose to or may be associated with subclinical DIC that may evolve into a massive postpartum haemorrhage. In such a situation, the coagulation profile should be tested and the abnormalities corrected with appropriate components before the process of delivery. Amniotic fluid embolism can result in acute fulminant DIC and bleeding. Therefore, one must empirically transfuse fresh frozen plasma, cryoprecipitate, and platelet units until further guidance is available with laboratory values.

Role of heparin/antifibrinolytics: Each of them has a role in the ongoing DIC if given at the correct time weighing the balance of excessive bleed/thrombosis in the given case. Removing the underlying cause of DIC should take priority along with supportive treatment. Antifibrinolytics can aggravate thrombosis, and heparin can exacerbate bleeding. In subclinical or chronic DIC in the thrombotic phase, heparin has a definite role. So, in women with florid sepsis or thrombotic manifestation or predisposition as occurs in a woman with thrombophilia and severe preeclampsia, heparin should be used, but in established acute fulminant DIC with bleeding, heparin has not been shown to have a role.

So, to summarise
1. Massive transfusion protocol should be followed as described in the previous chapter to prevent coagulopathy in the event of haemorrhage.
2. Women with known coagulation disorder should be kept under close surveillance, and the specific factors checked and corrected before anticipated delivery.
3. Women on anticoagulation should be switched over from Coumarin derivatives to heparin before delivery to minimise the haemorrhage-related complications.
4. One should expedite correction of the underlying obstetric cause for DIC, including delivery.
5. The other precautions are perfect haemostasis while suturing episiotomy.
6. One should avoid ventouse delivery in women on anticoagulants to minimise the fetus's known or unknown bleeding risk.
7. Consider placing an intraperitoneal and subcutaneous drain in women undergoing caesarean before complete correction of coagulation abnormality.

REFERENCES

1. Bakri YN. Balloon device for control of obstetrical bleeding. *Eur J Obstet Gynecol Reprod Biol.* 1999;86:S84.
2. Frenzel D, Condous GS, Papageorghiou AT, McWhinney NA. The use of the 'tamponade test' to stop massive obstetric haemorrhage in placenta accreta. *BJOG.* 2005;112:676–7.
3. Purwosunu Y, Sarkoen W, Arulkumaran S, Segnitz J. Control of postpartum hemorrhage using vacuum-induced uterine tamponade. *Obstet Gynecol.* 2016;128:33–6.

4. Selçuk İ, Uzuner B, Boduç E, Baykuş Y, Akar B, Güngör T. Step-by-step ligation of the internal iliac artery. *J Turk Ger Gynecol Assoc.* 2019;20(2):123–128. doi:10.4274/jtgga.galenos.2018.2018.0124.
5. Sultan AH, Thakar R. Third and fourth degree tear.In: Sultan AH, Thakar R, Fenner DE, eds. *Perineal and anal sphincter trauma.* London: Springer-Verlag Limited, 2007:34–40.
6. Sultan AH. Primary repair of obstetric anal sphincter injury. In: Staskin D, Cardozo L, eds. *Textbook of female urology and urogynaecology.* London: ISIS Medical Media, 2006 (in press).

FURTHER READING

Patil V, Shetmahajan M. Massive transfusion and massive transfusion protocol. *Indian J Anaesth.* 2014;58(5):590–595. doi:10.4103/0019-5049.144662.

Index

Note: *Italic* page numbers refer to figures.

abdominal examination 44–46, 52, 53, 61, 165
abnormal fetal heart rate pattern 113–114
abnormal uterine contractions 89–90
    abdominal rescue 125
    classification of 95–96
    complications of 103
    constriction ring 97
    management goals 101–103
    normal polarity 97–99
    oxytocin 99–100
    spastic lower uterine segment 97
    tetanic uterine contractions 96–97
    timeline definitions 100–101
absorbable suture 172
active management of the third stage of labour (AMTSL) 63, 159, 160
active phase, labour 33, 59–60
    definition of 59
    labour progress 60
    maternal condition 60
acupuncture 71
acute hypoxia 81
adult epidural needle 74
Alexandria unit 39
anaesthesia 54, 69, 97, 127, 145, 164, 174
anatomical conjugate 15
anatomical outlet 17, *18*
android pelvis 19–20
annular tears 173
anterior asynclitism 92
anterior episiotomy 65
anterior fontanella/bregma 27
anterior-posterior diameter 15–16, 17, 19, 23
anterior shoulder 151
anthropoid pelvis 22
antibiotics 154
anticoagulation 178
apes, pelvic ring 2
arcuate pubic ligament 10
arterial blood gas analysis (ABG) 163
arteriovenous malformation (AVM) 176
artificial rupture of membranes (ARM) 102, 112
aseptic technique 74
assimilation pelvis 110
asynclitism 91
atonic uterus 169–171, *170*
auscultation 46

baby weight 46, 53
bad obstetric outcome 111
Bakri Balloon 170
Bandl's ring 121
big baby 87, 117
bimastoid diameter 29
biparietal diameter 29
birth canal formation 34

bitemporal diameter 29
blade, forceps delivery 129
blood loss 158
blood pressure 58
blood replacement 162
breech presentation 41
bregma
    clinical significance of 27
    posterior fontanelle/lambda 27–28
broad ligament hematoma 153, 166
brow 29
bucket handle tear 173
bupivacaine 75

caesarean section
    classical caesarean section 144
    disadvantages 145
    fetal indications 143
    maternal indication 143
    for placenta previa 150
    preoperative preparations 144
    skin incision and steps 145
    steps of 146–147
    for transverse lie 150
    troubled situations 152
    various techniques 147
calmodulin calcium complex 38
caput formation 90
caput succidenum 91
cardiotocography (CTG) 77–79, *78*, 80, 81
cascade 83
case scenario partogram *57*
catecholamine surge 82
central organ oxygenation 82
central venous line 163
cephalic application 132
cephalic presentation 41, *42–43*
cephalopelvic disproportion (CPD)
    clinical identification tests 105–106
    contracted pelvis 107–108
    CT scan AND MRI, role of 107
    X-ray pelvimetry 107
cervical caput 91
cervical dystocia 98
cervix dilation 52
cervix, exploration of 165, *166*
Chassar Moir method 105
chemo-baroreceptor decelerations 83
childbirth 2
    anaesthesia for 69
    normal labour 31
choice, treatment of 96
chorioamnionitis 88
chronic hypoxia 82
classical caesarean section 144

classification of 64
cleidotomy 125
clinical pelvic assessment 16
clinical picture 82
coagulopathy 177–178
Cochrane Review (2015) 84
combined spinal epidural (CSE) 75
communication 163
complete anterior rotation 49
complications and management 76, 141
conjugates 15
Consortium of Labour 59
constriction ring (Schroeder's ring) 97–98
continuous epidural infusion (CEI) 76
contracted pelvis
    causes for 108
    congenital deformities 110–111
    inlet contraction 108
    midpelvic contraction 108
    objective definition for 108
    outlet contraction 108
    pelvis and joints 109–110
    spine, abnormalities of 109
    trial of labour 111
contraindications 74
coxa profunda 12
Crede's method 63
cryoprecipitate 162
8C's approach 82
cumulative uterine activity 82
cyclic adenosine monophosphate (cAMP) 38
cycling of FHR 82

Dare's formula 46
deceleration phase 33
deep transverse arrest (DTA) 49, 50, 117
    forceps extraction 118, 119
    management of 118
    manual rotation 118, *119*
    risk factors for 117
deflexed head 88
dehydration, correction of 101
delayed labour 84
delivery as head 151
delivery, shoulders *62*
denominator 41
diagnosis 123
diagonal conjugate 15, *16*
digital examination 164
digital rectal examination 66–67
Donald's method 106
Doppler method 78
Dublin protocol 100
dynamic longitudinal diameters 29
dysfunctional labour 88
dysfunctional uterine contractions 89

electromyography 39
Elliot's forceps 129
elytrotomy 153–154
emotional support 101
engagement diameter 41, 49
entonox cylinder 72
epidural analgesia 74

epidural catheters fixation 74
epidural hematoma 76
episiotomy 133
    anterior episiotomy 65
    caution word 67
    classification of 64
    digital rectal examination 66–67
    episiotomy scissors 65
    episiotomy side 65
    J-shaped 65
    mediolateral 65
    midline/median 64–65
    repair of episiotomy 65–66
episiotomy apex 174
episiotomy scissors 65
episiotomy side 65
evidence-based approach 39
excessive backache 89
extended head diameter 29
external conjugate 107
external pelvimetry 23–25, 106–107
external tocodynamometer 38–39

face 29
face to pubis delivery 120, *120*
failed forceps 134
falciform process 9
false/greater pelvis 5
false labour pain 51
fentanyl 73
fetal blood sampling (FBS) 84
fetal complications 141–142
    cephalhaematoma 141–142
    subgaleal hematoma 142
fetal compromise, risk factors 78
fetal concerns 123
fetal electrocardiography 84
fetal heart rate (FHR) 80, 82
fetal heart sounds 46, 53
fetal journey
    abdominal examination 44–46
    definitions and terminologies 41–44
    labour mechanism 46–50
    lie, fetus longitudinal axis 41, *42–43*
fetal physiology 77
fetal pillow device 152
fetal position 44–45
fetal scalp stimulation 84
fetal skull 27
    diameters of 29
    engagement of 29–30
    presenting part 41
FIGO Intrapartum Expert Consensus panel 81
first pelvic grip (Pawlik's grip) 45
first stage, labour 36
    active phase 33
    bag of membranes, formation 32
    cervix, dilatation and effacement 31–32
    descent of head 33
    fetal axis pressure 32–33
    latent phase 33, 36
    management
        admission 54
        ambulation and position 54

antibiotics 55
birth companion 55
diet and nutrition 54
dilation graph 58–59
emotional support 55
hospital policy 54
monitoring 55–58
pain relief 55
part preparation 54
mechanism 32
fish, pelvic ring 1
flexion point 139
floor muscles 6, 7
fluid replacement 161
fontanelles 27
forceps delivery
application 131–132
cephalic application 132
episiotomy 133
failed forceps 134
forceps, parts of 129–130
maternal exhaustion 132
mechanism of 131
pathological cardiotocograph 132
pelvic application 132
perineal support 134
procedure 132–133
prophylactic application 132
rotation and extraction 135
trial of forceps 132
ventouse delivery 142
forceps rotation 119
free-floating head 149
fresh frozen plasma (FFP) transfusion 162
full hand method 118, *119*
fundal height 44
funic souffle 46

glabella 28
greater pelvis 5
growth, pelvis 3–4
gynecoid pelvis 19

Hadlock's formula 46
half hand method 118, *119*
halogenated agents 72
handles, forceps delivery 129
head, coning of 90, 91
head descent, labour 33, 100
failure/arrest of 100–101
health care system 54
HELLP (Hemolysis elevated liver enzyme and low
platelet) syndrome 159
heparin/antifibrinolytics role 178
hip morphology 2
hyperstimulation 98
hypnosis 71
hypotension 76
hypoxic ischaemic encephalopathy (HIE) 77

ideal maintenance technique 75–76
iliolumbar ligament 9
immersion in water 71
incomplete anterior rotation 50

incoordinate uterine contractions 96
indications 73
inhalational methods 72
inlet/superior pelvic aperture 5, 15, 108
antero-posterior diameter 15–16
boundaries of 15
sacro-cotyloid diameter 16–17
transverse diameter 16
intensity 37
intermittent auscultation 78, 80
internal examination 53
internal iliac artery ligation 172
internal podalic version 127–128
internal rotation 47
internal uterine pressure 39
interpubic disc 10
intra-abdominal pressure 38
intrapartum fetal surveillance
adjunctive technologies 83–84
cardiotocography 77–79
fetal compromise, risk factors 78
fetal physiology 77
intermittent auscultation 78
intrapartum surveillance method 78
intrauterine resuscitation concept 83
intrapartum surveillance method 78
intrapartum ultrasound 84
intra-pelvic adaptations 2
intrauterine pressure 37
intrauterine resuscitation concept 83

JADA device 171
Joel-Cohen technique 147
Johnson's formula 46
"J"- shaped curve 18, 65

Kielland forceps 119, 129, *130,* 135
kiwi cups 137, 139
kyphosis 109

labour
active phase of 90, 100
affecting factors 36
augmentation of 88
fetal position 44–45
first stage of 31–33
fourth stage of 35–36
LOA position 47
management
active labour 59–60
episiotomy 64–67
false labour pain 51
first stage 54–58
labour graph progress
58–59
labour signs 51–52
risk assessment 52
second stage 60–62
symptoms 51
third stage 63–64
woman examination 52–54
mechanism of *48*
pelvic assessment 22, *24–25*
pudendal nerve block 9

labour (*cont.*)
    second stage of 33–34
    third stage of 35
labour epidural initiation 75
labour pain
    somatic pain 70
    visceral pain 70
lamaze breathing technique 71
Lamberting technique 148
LaQshyya guidelines 55
latent phase, labour 33
lateral extension 152
lateral flexion 47
lateral grips 44–45
left occipito-anterior (LOA) 44
left occipito-posterior (LOP) 44
left occipito-transverse (LOT) 44
Leopold's grips 53
lesser pelvis 5, 6
lie, fetus longitudinal axis 41, *42–43*
linear tears 173
linea terminalis 4
liquor, clinical assessment 53
LOA position 47
local anaesthetic agents 75
lock, forceps delivery 130
longitudinal ovoid 27
loss of resistance (LOR) technique 74
lower segment 37, 39
    anatomical identification 39
    clinical importance 39

male and female pelvis bones 11–12
malformations 87
malposition 87
malpresentations 88
massage 71
massive blood transfusion 176–177
massive transfusion protocol 177
maternal complications 141
maternal condition 60
maternal dehydration 89
maternal exhaustion 132
maternal passage
    clinical pelvimetry 22–25
    pelvis
        android pelvis 19–22
        anthropoid pelvis 22
        carus, curve of *16*, 18
        clinical application and diameter 15–17
        gynecoid pelvis 19
        least pelvic dimensions 18–19
        mid pelvic cavity 17
        outlet of pelvis 17–18
        platypelloid pelvis 22
maternal request 73
maternal stress response 88
maternal tachycardia 89
Mathew Duncan method 35
McRoberts manoeuvre 123–124, *125*
mechanism, pelvis 12–13
meconium-stained liquor 88–89, 97
mediolateral 65
mentovertical diameter 29
mentum 28

meperidine (pethidine) 73
metal cup 137, 139
midline/median 64–65
mid pelvic cavity 17
midpelvic contraction 108
Misgav Ladach technique 147
Montevideo units 37, 39
morphine 73
moulding 90–91
mucus plug expulsion 51
Muller-Kerr method 106
multiple gestations 88
multiple pregnancies 126–127
    internal podalic version 127–128
musculo-fascial pelvic diaphragm 5
myosin protein 38

Naegel's obliquity 92
nasion 28
neuraxial techniques
    combined spinal epidural 75
    complications and management 76
    contraindications 74
    epidural analgesia 74
    ideal maintenance technique 75–76
    indications 73
NICE guidelines 144
non-pharmacological methods 71
normal labour
    definition of 31
    fetal skull 27
normal polarity
    cervical dystocia 98
    precipitate labour 98
    uterine inertia 97–98
    uterine tachysystole 98
normal uterine contractions 37, *96*
normeperidine 73
nutrition 101
nutritional disorders 109

obesity 87
oblique diameter 17
obstetric analgesia
    history 69
    labour pain 70
    neuraxial techniques
        combined spinal epidural 75
        complications and management 76
        contraindications 74
        epidural analgesia 74
        ideal maintenance technique 75–76
        indications 73
    non-pharmacological methods 71
    pain pathway 70
    pharmacological methods 71
        inhalational methods 72
        parenteral opioids 73
obstetric conjugate 15
obstetric factors 178
obstetric outlet 17
obstructed labour 121
    clinical features 121–122
    fate of obstructed labour 122
    pathophysiology of 121

prevention of 122
treatment of 122–123
occipito-frontal diameter 29
occipito-posterior positions 44, 47–48
occipito-transverse position 45
occiput 28
oligohydramnios 117
opioid addition 75
ossification 4
osteomalacia 110
outlet contraction 108
outlet/inferior pelvic aperture 6
outlet of pelvis
anatomical outlet 17, 18
obstetric outlet 17
overzealous perfusion 177
oxygen 161
oxytocin
Dublin protocol 100
regimens of 99–100
oxytocin augmentation 102, 122

pacemakers 37
pain pathway 70
pain relief 101
palpation 44
parenteral opioids 73
pathological cardiotocograph 132
patient-controlled epidural analgesia (PCEA) 76
Patwardhan technique 151
pelvic application 132
pelvic assessment 22, 24–25
pelvic brim index 5, 10
pelvic caput 91
pelvis anatomy
anatomical position 7
axis and inclination 7
evolution 1–3
female and male pelvis shape 12
floor muscles actions 7
greater/false pelvis 5
infancy to adulthood 3–4
inlet/superior pelvic aperture 5
joints and ligaments 4
iliolumbar ligament 9
pubic symphysis 10
sacrococcygeal joint 10
sacroiliac joint 7
sacroiliac ligaments 7–8
sacrospinous ligament 9
sacrotuberous ligament 8–9
lesser pelvis 5, 6
mechanism 12–13
morphological classification 10–11
outlet/inferior pelvic aperture 6
pelvic floor 6
pelvic walls 4–5
sexual differences 11–12
perineal support 134, 141
persistent asynclitism 90
persistent deflexed head 117
persistent occipito-posterior position 50
pfannenstiel incision 145, 147
pharmacological methods 71
inhalational methods 72

parenteral opioids 73
physical examination 52
Pinard's method 106
placental separation 35, 35
placenta, manual removal 175
placenta previa 150
plane, least pelvic dimensions 17
compensatory diameters 19
importance of 18–19
transverse diameter 19
platelets 162
platypelloid pelvis 22
pocket tears 173–174
polarity 37
polyhydramnios 88
poor Bishop Score 88
post-dural puncture headache (PDPH) 76
posterior asynclitism 92
posterior sagittal diameter (PSD) 23
postoperative care 154
post-partum haemorrhage (PPH)
classification 158
clinical approach
definitive management 164–167
effective resuscitation 161–163
initial management 163–164
clinical identification 157–158
definitions of 157
management
atonic uterus 169–171
coagulopathy 177–178
massive blood transfusion 176–177
retained products 174–175
secondary postpartum haemorrhage 175–176
stepwise surgical devascularisation 171–173
traumatic, management of 173–174
postoperative care of 175
PPH, prevention of 159–160
predisposing factors 158–159
post-term pregnancy 88
precipitate labour 98
predict labour dystocia 39
predisposing factors 87
pregnancy, screening in 177
prelabour 51
premature bearing down 89
prematurity 140
prerequisites 140
presentation 41
presenting part 41
preventing infection 112
primary cervical dystocia 98
primigravid woman 33
programmed intermittent epidural boluses (PIEB) 76
prolonged latent phase 95, 100
prophylactic application 132
proteins/ketones 58
protracted dilation 100
pruritus 76
pubic symphysis 10, 17
pull
direction of 131
do's and don'ts 133–134
ventouse delivery 140–141
pulse 58

Purandare's method 106
push method 34, 151; *see also* pull

rachitic pelvis 109
recombinant factor VIIa (rFVIIa) 163
remifentanil 73
repair of episiotomy 65–66
rescue plan 141
restitution 47
retraction 37
reverse breech method 151
reverse Wood corkscrew 124
risk assessment 52
Robson's classification 144
ropivacaine 75
Rubin I manoeuvre 124

sacrococcygeal joint 10
sacro-cotyloid diameter 16
sacroiliac joint 7
sacroiliac ligaments 7–8
sacrospinous ligament 9
sacrotuberous ligament 8–9
Schultze's method 35
secondary postpartum haemorrhage 175–176
second pelvic grip 45–46
second stage, labour 33–34
    abnormalities
        arrest in, labour 115–117
        deep transverse arrest 117
    delivery, conduct of 61
    identification 60–61
    maternal and fetal monitoring 61
    modified ritgen manoeuvre 61–62
separation Schultze's method 35
sexual dimorphism 11
shank, forceps delivery 129
The shortening myofibril 32
shoulder dystocia 123
    complications of 126
    McRoberts manoeuvre 123–124, *125*
    prevention of 126
    reverse Wood corkscrew 124
    Rubin I manoeuvre 124
    Woods Corkscrew manoeuvre 124
    Zavanelli manoeuvre 125
silastic cup 137, 139
Simpsons forceps 129
sinciput 28
skin incision 149
Snow, John Dr. 69
somatic pain 70
spastic lower uterine segment 97
spondylolisthesis 109
spontaneous labour lack 88
spontaneous short posterior rotation 49–50
static diameters 29
ST wave analysis (STAN) 84
subacute hypoxia 81
submentobregmatic diameter 29
submentovertical diameter 29
sub-mentum 28
suboccipito-bregmatic diameter 29
suboccipito-frontal diameter 29

sub-occiput 28
subpubic angle 18
suction apparatus 139
suction tubing 138
Sultan Classification 174
super-sub parietal diameter 29
supine hypotension 79
suprapubic bulge 35
surgical intervention, principles of 171
symphysio-fundal height 44
symphysiotomy 125
synclitism 91

tachyphylaxis 99
tears involving fornix 174
tetanic uterine contractions 96–97
third stage, labour 35
    components, AMTSL 64
    controlled cord traction 63
    placental delivery, conduct of 63
    uterotonic agents, AMTSL 64
thromboprophylaxis 154
tone, basal intrauterine pressure 38
traditional surgical options 171
transcutaneous electrical nerve stimulation (TENS) 71
transition phase 33
transverse diameter 16, 17, 19
transverse ovoid 27
trauma, predisposing factors for 159
trial labour
    abnormal fetal heart rate pattern 113–114
    adequate hydration and nutrition 113
    analgesia 113
    artificial rupture of membranes 112
    delivery mode 113
    endpoint of 113
    labour, augmentation of 112
    management of 111–114
    uterus, secondary inertia of 113
trial of forceps 132
true conjugate 15
true labour pains 51
true pelvis 4, 5
    inlet, clinical significance 16–17
turtle sign 123

ultrasound assessment 46
universal flexion attitude 41
upper segment 40
urinary bladder, catheterisation 150
urinary catheter 161
uterine activity
    electromyography 39
    external tocodynamometer 38–39
    internal uterine pressure 39
    measurement of 38
uterine artery clamp 171
uterine artery ligature 172
uterine contractions 33, 34, 51–52
    biomolecular basis 38
    coordination 38
    intensity 37
    pacemakers 37
    polarity 37

retraction 37
    synchrony 38
uterine incision 149
uterine inertia 97–98
uterine myofibril
    retraction 37
uterine segments
    formation of 39
    lower segment 39
    upper segment 40
uterine souffle 46
uterine tachysystole 98
uterus, malformations of 88

vaginal examination 27, 60
vaginal hematomas 167
vaginal tears 173
vault/cranium 27, *28*
    anterior fontanella/bregma 27
    fontanelles 27
ventouse cup 137
ventouse delivery
    apparatus for 137–139
    application and pull 140–141
    complications 141
    fetal complications 141–142
    forceps-assisted deliveries 142
    mechanism of 139–140
ventouse rotation 120
vertex 28
    presentations 29, *44,* 149
vertical extension 153
vertical incision 145
visceral pain 70
voided urine volume 58
vulvo-vaginal hematomas 167

waterblocks 71
woman, during labour
    abdominal examination 52
    in active labour 58
    on anticoagulants 140
    internal examination 53
    pelvic assessment 53
    physical examination 52
    true labour pains 51
    uterine contractions 51–52
Woods Corkscrew manoeuvre 124
World Health Organization (WHO) *56,* 58, 64, 160
Wrigley's outlet forceps 129, *130*

Zavanelli manoeuvre 125

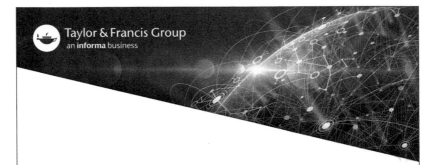